Introducing the Social Sciences for Midwifery Practice

Introducing the Social Sciences for Midwifery Practice makes clear the links between social, anthropological and psychological concepts, midwifery practice and women's experience of birth. Demonstrating how empathising with women and understanding the context in which they live can affect childbirth outcomes and experiences, this evidence-based text emphasises the importance of compassionate and humane care in midwifery practice.

Exploring midwifery as an art, as well as a science, the authors collected here make the case for midwives as professionals working 'with women' rather than as birth technicians, taking a purely competency-based approach to practice. The book incorporates a range of pedagogical features to enhance student learning, including overall chapter aims and learning outcomes, 'recommendations for practice', 'learning triggers' to encourage the reader to delve deeper and reflect on practice, 'application to practice' case studies that ensure that the theory is related to contemporary practice, and a glossary of terms. The chapters cover perspectives on birth from sociology, psychology, anthropology, law, social policy and politics. Other chapters address important issues such as disability and sexuality.

Outlining relevant theory from the social sciences and clearly applying it to practice, this text is an essential read for all student midwives, registered midwives and doulas.

Patricia Lindsay did her nurse training in London, then trained as a midwife. She has been a practising midwife since 1974, and a midwifery teacher since 1991. She has worked in the UK and in the Sultanate of Oman. She was Lead Midwife for Education at Anglia Ruskin University, UK, until the end of August 2014. Her doctoral thesis was on incident reporting in maternity care and she has presented posters on this topic at national and international conferences. Her interests are patient safety in maternity care, women's mental health and support-worker training.

Ian Peate began his nursing career in 1981 at Central Middlesex Hospital, becoming an enrolled nurse working in an intensive care unit. He later undertook three years of student nurse training at Central Middlesex and Northwick Park Hospitals, becoming a staff nurse, then a charge nurse. He has worked in nurse education since 1989. His key areas of interest are nursing practice and theory, men's health, sexual health and HIV. Ian has published widely; he is Professor of Nursing and Head of School, School of Health Studies Gibraltar and Editor in Chief, *British Journal of Nursing*.

Introducing the Social Sciences for Midwifery Practice

Birthing in a contemporary society

Edited by Patricia Lindsay and Ian Peate

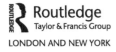
Routledge
Taylor & Francis Group

LONDON AND NEW YORK

First published 2016
by Routledge
2 Park Square, Milton Park, Abingdon, Oxon OX14 4RN

and by Routledge
711 Third Avenue, New York, NY 10017

Routledge is an imprint of the Taylor & Francis Group, an informa business

British Library Cataloguing-in-Publication Data
A catalogue record for this book is available from the British Library

Library of Congress Cataloging in Publication Data
Introducing the social sciences for midwifery practice : birthing in a contemporary society / edited by Patricia Lindsay and Ian Peate.
    p. ; cm.
  Includes bibliographical references and index.
  I. Lindsay, Patricia, 1951–, editor.   II. Peate, Ian, editor.
  [DNLM: 1. Midwifery—methods.   2. Sociological Factors.
  3. Sociology, Medical. WQ 160]
  RG950
  618.2—dc23   2014048872

ISBN: 978-1-138-01553-1 (hbk)
ISBN: 978-1-138-01554-8 (pbk)
ISBN: 978-1-315-79428-0 (ebk)

Typeset in Sabon
by Keystroke, Station Road, Codsall, Wolverhampton

Dedication

This book is dedicated to the women and families
we care for and who teach midwives most of what they know.

Contents

List of figures, tables and boxes

Figures

Tables

Boxes

Author biographies

Andy Alaszewski is Emeritus Professor of Health Studies at the University of Kent. He is an applied social scientist who has examined the ways in which social policy making has shaped the ways in health and social care professionals deliver health and social care. He edits *Health, Risk & Society*, an international peer reviewed journal, and is author of *Using Diaries for Social Research* 2006 and co-author of *Risk, Safety and Clinical Practice: Healthcare through the lens of risk 2010* (with B. Heyman and colleagues) and *Making Health Policy: A Critical Introduction 2012* (with Patrick Brown).

Christine Grabowska RN, RM, BSc, MSc, ADM, PGCEA, Lic Ac, Lic OHM, Dip CST trained as a nurse at St George's and as a midwife at the Whittington Hospitals in London. She completed her BSc in the Social Sciences at the London School of Economics and her Master's in Medical Sociology at the Royal Holloway. She has worked with women supporting them in their births at home, hospital and in combination with the DOMINO scheme. She became a midwife teacher in 1990 and later became an acupuncturist, oriental herbalist and cranio-sacral therapist. Her research looked at combining midwifery with traditional Chinese medicine, pursuing the use of moxibustion to turn a breech presentation. She teaches the social sciences and has further interests in human rights, physiological birth and nurturing.

Louise Hunter PhD, MA (Oxon), RM studied theology at Oxford before training to be a midwife in 1999, after the births of her two children. She has worked as a community midwife in Oxford and as a lecturer at the University of West London, and is now a senior lecturer in midwifery at Oxford Brookes University. Louise's doctoral thesis on young mothers and breastfeeding led her to examine the culture of the postnatal ward and its impact on care and maternal wellbeing.

Patricia Lindsay RN, RM, MSc, PGCEA, DHC did her nurse training in London and then trained as a midwife. She has been a practising midwife since 1974, and a midwifery teacher since 1991. She has worked in the UK and in the Sultanate of Oman. She was Lead Midwife for Education at Anglia Ruskin University until the end of August 2014. Her doctoral thesis was on incident reporting in maternity care and she has presented posters on this topic at national and international conferences. Her interests are patient safety in maternity care, women's mental health and support worker training.

Kate Nash RGN, RM, BSc (Hons), MSc trained and practiced as a general nurse in London before undertaking her midwifery training in 1998. She has worked in both community and high-dependency maternity settings in various roles within London, the Midlands and southeast England. She completed her teaching training in 2007 and is employed as a senior lecturer in midwifery at the University of West London. Kate has worked as a Supervisor of Midwives (SOM) since 2009 and is currently a member of the SOM team at Frimley Health NHS Foundation Trust (Wexham Park Hospital). She is undertaking her clinical doctorate, investigating midwifery practice during the second stage of labour. Her key areas of interest also include complicated childbirth, birth emergencies, professional issues and the broader sociological issues that impact upon midwifery practice and maternity care.

Elizabeth Prochaska BA, LLB, BCL is a barrister at Matrix Chambers in London, where she specialises in public and human rights law. She is the co-author of the *Blackstone Guide to the Human Rights Act 1998*. Since the birth of her daughter, she has regularly advised women and health professionals on the law relating to maternity care. In 2013, she founded Birthrights with fellow lawyers and health professionals to campaign for the respectful treatment of women in childbirth.

Mandie Scamell RM, PGCEA, BSc, MRes, MSc began her career in midwifery in Kent in 1995. Mandie has worked within a case-loading model of care and has specialised in high-risk pregnancy care. With a research background in medical anthropology, Mandie has been involved in UK maternity care research for several years publishing in *Midwifery*, *British Journal of Midwifery* and *Practising Midwives* as well as several other high-impact social science journals. Her current research interests are in how understandings of risk impact upon midwifery practice. Mandie is Midwifery Lecturer at City University London.

Caroline Squire RN, RM, ADM, PGCEA, MSc (Medical Anthropology), Lic Ac, Lic OHM, PGDip (Research Methods) trained as a midwife at The Olive Haydon School of Midwifery at St Thomas and Guy's maternity units qualifying in 1981. She became a community midwife in 1983 and was active in promoting home births and DOMINO births in an inner London practice. She became a lecturer in 1988 and worked at the University of West London until 2013, teaching predominantly from the social sciences as well as anatomy. Caroline is an acupuncturist and oriental herbalist and a reader for the British Acupuncture Accreditation Board. She has published widely and, currently, is editing the third edition of her book *The Social Context of Childbirth*, which will be published in 2016. Her key interests related to childbirth are social and economic inequalities in the UK, domestic abuse and birth following sexual abuse.

Mary Stewart RM, PhD has worked as a midwife for more than 30 years. Mary worked for many years as a community midwife, and has also worked as a midwifery lecturer. From 2007–2010 she was a research midwife working on the Birthplace Study at the National Perinatal Epidemiology Unit (NPEU), in Oxford. She now works as a research midwife at University College London, working on Life Study, a large longitudinal cohort study that aims to understand how the family, social and physical environment influence the health, development and wellbeing of babies and children.

Susan Walker MB BCh., BA (Hons.), MPhil, PhD started her career as a general practitioner and developed an interest in women's health and in the sociological aspects of health. After completing a PhD at the University of Cambridge she took up a post as Senior Lecturer in Sexual Health at Anglia Ruskin University. Her doctoral thesis explored the effect of gendered body image on contraceptive outcomes. Her interests include the effects of gender and sexuality upon health behaviours, and her research interests lie at the intersection of sociology and medicine.

Maxine Wallis-Redworth RN, RM, BSc, MSc, PGCEA, IBCLC trained as a nurse in New Zealand before coming to England to train as a midwife. She has been a practising midwife since 1982 and has worked in education in the UK since 1990. Her primary interest is lactation management and she qualified as an International Board Certified Lactation Consultant in 2009. She is a Course leader for the BSc (Hons) Midwifery Course at Anglia Ruskin University and works clinically as part of a Cambridge breastfeeding drop-in clinic team. She is undertaking a professional doctorate at the University of Central Lancashire, focusing on breastfeeding self-efficacy related to fathers.

Jane Weaver RN, RM, PhD, PGDip began nurse training in London in 1972, followed by midwifery training in Cumbria. She practised as a midwife in Cumbria, then as a RAF nursing sister (PMRAFNS), followed by a post as a staff midwife, then as a community midwifery sister in Huntingdon. She then took a break from midwifery to read for a BSc in Psychology, followed by a PhD, both at University College London. After three and a half years research at Cambridge University she returned to midwifery education, eventually becoming Professor of Midwifery at the University of West London before her retirement in 2013. Jane's research interests have included choice and control in childbirth, decision making for caesarean section and media representation of childbearing women.

Acknowledgements

Pat would like to thank her husband Paul for his continuing support and care.

Ian would like to thank his partner Jussi Lahtinen for his ongoing support and encouragement.

Preface

This text draws on a number of theories in order to elaborate on the care that midwives offer women and their families as well as the work of the midwife in constantly changing environments. It provides the reader with an introduction to psycho-social, legal and political aspects of maternity care, shedding light on and assisting with policy development. The book balances the current largely skill and competence-driven approach to midwifery practice with insights into social theory and the social and political structures within which this approach has arisen.

The text has been written with the student midwife in mind, however, others (for example, the registered midwife) may find the contents of value assisting them in their pursuit to offer women and their families care that focuses on their holistic needs.

Sandall (2014) highlights the need for midwife-led continuity models to include an emphasis on the natural ability of women to experience birth with minimum intervention and to monitor the physical, psychological, spiritual and social wellbeing of the woman and family during the childbearing cycle. This unique book provides the reader with an overview of the social influences (the social sciences) that can impact on women and birthing in relation to the art and science of midwifery practice. In this one text readers are able to access contemporary information, debates and discussions concerning fundamental issues pertaining to childbearing that may be overlooked in other midwifery texts.

This approach negates the need for the reader to have to access other texts and then go back and apply the social influences to their practice; the contributors provide the reader with all of the information in one place. In reality many students may never access texts on these important issues that have impacted on and influenced midwifery practice. By using this book the reader has all of the pertinent information at their fingertips.

For the first time this book brings together discussion concerning the social sciences (i.e. sociology, psychology and anthropology) and how this relates to contemporary midwifery practice, it clarifies the recent proposed reforms outlined in the Francis Inquiry (2013) and Keogh Review (National Health Service, 2013).

There are chapters on choice and consent in childbirth, the concepts of labelling and deviance in childbirth, spirituality and childbirth, all of which impact on compassionate and courageous care. The chapters are steeped in social science theory with application to the woman, birthing and society and they are written by midwives who have wealth of experience in practice and academia. The chapter on sociology, for example, outlines the key sociological theories and the author uses these theories, applying them to contemporary midwifery practice. The chapter on psychology is another example of how psychological theory is influential in the provision of safe, appropriate high-quality care to women and their families.

Contributors are practising midwives who believe that an understanding of these key concepts is essential to how midwives conceptualise their roles and how women receive midwifery care. Current midwifery curricula lack the overt application to and linking with the social issues that impact on the woman and childbirth that should underpin our understanding of society and therefore the place of women and midwives within it. Without this knowledge students and midwives will be limited in their understanding of their role and how they can work within societal constraints to achieve a satisfying experience for the women and themselves.

It is acknowledged that the work of the midwife is becoming increasingly technical, reflecting midwifery as a science rather than an art. Midwives are taking on an ever-more technical and bureaucratic workload. This has the potential to reconstruct their role as that of birth technician, rather than a professional who is 'with woman'.

One of the overarching aims of this book is to start a change, as there are concerns that midwives may be becoming emotionally distant, while women's birth stories demonstrate a great need for a more humanitarian approach to their care. This need is reflected in the increasing numbers of women traumatised by a mechanical approach to care that does not understand the social context of the birth experience.

We use a variety of approaches to engage the reader, for example, we have included 'triggers' to help students grow and develop their practise, to delve deeper and generate a sense of curiosity, and 'application to practice' features are included in order to bring alive the subject area as well as helping the student apply this to their practice. A glossary of terms is provided. The chapters offer fundamental information relevant to midwifery and maternity care generally, interspersed with activities helping readers to make links between the topic and what she/he is learning from both practice and academic experience. This will enhance learning, help close the theory–practice gap and humanise maternity care.

We have enjoyed writing this text and we sincerely hope you enjoy reading and learning from it, with the express intention of responding to the needs of women and their families in a humanistic and woman-centred way.

References

Francis, R. (2013) *The Francis Report. The Report of the Mid Staffordshire NHS Foundation Trust Public Inquiry*. Online at: www.midstaffspublicinquiry.com/sites/default/files/report/ Executive summary.pdf, last accessed October 2014

National Health Service (2013) *Review into the Quality of Care and Treatment Provided by 14 Hospital Trusts in England: Overview Report*. Online at: www.nhs.uk/

NHSEngland/bruce-keogh-review/Documents/outcomes/keogh-review-final-report.pdf, last accessed October 2014

Sandall, J. (2014) *The Contribution of Continuity of Midwifery Care to High Quality Maternity Care*. Royal College of Midwives, London

Foreword

Why is it important for those involved in the planning and delivery of services for pregnant and childbearing women and their children to know what the social sciences can offer? Because reproduction and childbearing are transformational social and life events of interest to every society around the globe, because although the physiological process of childbearing has some universal characteristics, the way pregnancy and birth is managed varies widely around the world. 'Maternity care is a 'highly charged mix of medical science, cultural ideas and structural forces' (De Vries et al. 2001), and are so much more than a clinical episode.

Reproduction and childbearing have social and political dimensions, and the way that childbearing women are treated is a lens into how a society values women. The empowerment of women is the most important influence on maternal and infant morbidity and mortality around the globe. How a society chooses to spend or not spend its money on supporting childbearing women and families has an immediate effect on what services are provided, whether midwives are employed at all, and has a profound effect on clinical outcomes.

The social sciences can offer an insight into the relationship between wider society and the individual, into individual and organisational behaviour, and into the political economy of health care. They provide an important understanding as to how inequalities in income and wealth distribution at a country level have a more powerful effect than health services on morbidity and mortality.

The social sciences also provide an understanding and insight into knowledge production and the politics of knowledge. Claims over who has specialist knowledge and expertise have been integral to the successful establishment of occupations such as medicine and midwifery. As a student midwife in the 1970s, we were not allowed access to medical libraries to access journals without a letter from a doctor. The democratisation of knowledge through the internet and the synthesis of knowledge which is the foundation of evidence-based healthcare has enabled other occupations such as midwifery and the public to challenge and make their own decisions.

So to sum up, the main contribution of the social sciences is that they provide another way of looking at the world and the tools to help us understand and analyse why and how things are as they are. Most importantly they help us understand how change has occurred and what the critical factors are that need to be in place for change to happen in the future.

The chapters in this book provide an insight into how different social science disciplines focus on different levels of analysis and how such concepts can be applied to understanding the development of midwifery as a profession, policy formation, and how power needs to be taken into account in relationships between providers and women. Studies of women with disability and of sexuality in childbirth can also provide a lens to look at underlying attitudes and culture.

Jane Sandall
Professor of Social Science and Women's Health
Division of Women's Health Faculty of Life Sciences & Medicine,
King's College London,
Women's Health Academic Centre, St. Thomas' Hospital
London

Reference

De Vries, R. Benoit, C. Van Teijlingen, E. Wrede, S. (2001) *Birth by Design: Pregnancy, maternity care and midwifery in North America and Europe*, London, Routledge, p. xii.

1 Introduction to sociology

Kate Nash

Aim

The aim of this chapter is to offer an introduction to the subject of sociology and outline some of the main sociological theories and research methods used within sociological inquiry. It is hoped that through reading this chapter readers will begin to think more analytically about how societies function and consider the social influences that shape our own interpretations of the world and everyday social interactions.

Learning outcomes

By the end of the chapter the reader should be able to:

- Understand the relevance of sociology both as an academic discipline and its role in helping us to understand society today
- Explore the relevance of sociology for midwifery practice and theory
- Identify some of the main sociological theories
- Articulate some of the different theoretical approaches used within sociological research
- Summarise the key research methods used within sociological research
- Discuss the contribution of sociological research to midwifery knowledge

---

Introduction

As its name suggests the discipline of sociology involves the study of society and Giddens and Sutton (2013) define sociology as the scientific study of human social life, groups and societies. In particular, the British Sociological Association has emphasised how the study of sociology consists of trying to understand how society works by scrutinising different societies and the many forms of relationship that exist between groups and individuals both on a large and smaller scale (British Sociological Association, n.d.). It is through such scrutiny that we can appreciate how groups have formed and relationships established to provide the structure and **culture** within which we live and operate. This is generally acquired through the process of **socialisation** (Browne, 2011), which plays a vital part in how we form individual and group identities. Social control is the term given to the various methods used within societies to ensure that groups and individuals conform to established social values that have been learnt through socialisation. **Sanctions** are often used to achieve social control and both socialisation and social control help to maintain social order and ensure that groups conform to the expected codes and values of the group (Browne, 2011).

Trigger

Read *The Code: Professional Standards of Practice and Behaviour for Nurses and Midwives* (Nursing and Midwifery Council, NMC, 2015). Online at: www.nmc-uk.org/Publications/Standards/The-code/Introduction/

Consider the standards that govern the behaviour and conduct of nurses, midwives and health visitors. How are these standards enforced and what are the possible consequences (or sanctions) imposed for midwives failing to conform to these standards?

This chapter is divided into two sections. Section one provides an overview of the major sociological theories and perspectives, while section two summarises the various approaches and methods used within sociological research and considers the relevance of sociological research for midwives today.

There are many divisions and categories that exist within the study of sociology and Sharp (2010) describes sociology as being multi paradigmatic, meaning that it has been shaped over the years by many different perspectives and interpretations. It is impossible within the constraints of this chapter to do justice to the intricacies and complexities of sociological theory and so the reader is directed to a variety of resources throughout this chapter should they wish to develop their study further.

Being able to understand and engage with research and evidence-based practice forms a vital part of midwifery curricula within the United Kingdom today. Closely linked with sociological theory, sociological research seeks to inform us about society and many of the research methods used within healthcare today have their roots in sociological inquiry. The second section of this chapter presents an overview of the different approaches used by those undertaking sociological inquiry.

Overview of the main historical sociological theories

Structural theories

In order to understand sociology it is important to view the development of sociology theory against the emerging background which it evolved to provide context and enable an understanding of its importance and relevance at that time. The term 'sociology' was coined by the French philosopher Auguste Comte (1798–1857). Comte made reference to the term sociology in his 1822 publication 'Plan des travaux scientifiques nécessaires pour réorganiser la société' or 'terms of scientific work needed to reorganise society' and is believed by many to be one of the original founders of sociology.

Comte was born at the end of the French Revolution and a period of eighteenth-century European philosophy known as the Age of Enlightenment. This period was identified as an intellectual movement that encouraged and advocated scientific investigation and political philosophical debate as a way to create an influential system of ethics, aesthetics and knowledge. Comte put forward a considerable argument for the justification of sociology as an academic discipline and presented a law of three states whereby he believed that society must progress through three periods of intellectual development: theological, metaphysical and scientific. Comte believed that this progression was the principal cause of social change and that was also reflected within the scientific development apparent at that time.

Comte's philosophy subscribed very much to a positivist approach (Comte, 1854) and he proposed that the objective of positivism was to 'generalise our scientific conceptions and to systematise the art of social life' (Comte, 1854, p. 3). The traditional scientific or experimental approach to conducting research has its underpinnings in positivism (Robson, 2002) and positivists hold a fundamental belief in objective reality and the assumption that phenomena have antecedent causes (Polit and Beck, 2004). Comte argued that the study of sociology should be based on **empirical** evidence that was drawn from observation, comparison and experimentation and set out his proposal for a **scientific method** of organising experience.

Comte also suggested that society is a system whose parts are interconnected in ways that would have consequences for the maintenance of the social whole. **Structural theories** of society are described as having a **macro perspective**, whereby the focus is less on the specific actions of an individual but on the roles that they occupy and how these relate to each other and interconnect to form the whole (Sharp, 2010). When analysing roles the focus of structural theories is not on the individual occupying the roles but on the nature of the role itself and the expectations and standards expected by society of a particular role. This enables groups and organisations to be considered independently of the different people that constitute them (Sharp, 2010).

Trigger

Consider how midwives are viewed within society. You may wish to think about recent media coverage and terms used when describing midwives as a professional group. How might your own views of midwifery have changed since starting your midwifery training?

The two main structural theories are **functionalism** and **Marxism**. Functionalism is a branch of sociology that emphasises how different elements of society work harmoniously as a series of interconnected parts that together form a whole (Haralambos and Holborn, 2013). Social institutions such as the family are therefore analysed as a whole rather than as isolated components and it is believed that in order for such institutions to survive within society, there must be the fulfilment of necessary conditions of existence called functional prerequisites (Haralambos and Holborn, 2004). These functional prerequisites are based upon the socialisation of shared customs and values and various approaches have been used to identify what these are and the factors that different societies have in common. Thus functionalists focus on how social systems are maintained by the contribution of the specified prerequisites.

Functionalism became the dominant social theory within sociology up until the 1940s and 1950s and was developed by another French philosopher Émile Durkheim (1858–1917) who is widely regarded as one of the most influential functionalist theorists and important in establishing sociology as a serious academic discipline. Durkheim was active at a time when France was undergoing great social and economic upheaval and strove to consider how social groups could function together to form a cohesive society.

Often referred to as **consensus theory**, functionalism emphasises an essential consensus that should operate within societies and is particularly concerned with the maintenance of social order. Durkheim believed that the essence of human nature was twofold: partly driven by selfish desires and partly by an ability to believe in and adhere to moral values. By having a **collective conscience** comprising of shared beliefs and attitudes, Durkheim believed that it was possible for humans to become integrated into the dominant values of society and achieve social order. Like Comte, Durkheim adopted a positivist approach and focused upon the observable and the measurable as opposed to the internalised subjective experience.

Although Durkheim had little to say about healthcare, later functionalist sociologists sought to consider the various aspects of health and its management. Talcott Parsons (1902–1979) considered the concept of the sick role and argued that adhering to such a role helps to ensure the smooth running of society and ensure disruption is kept to a minimum. A criticism of the functionalist approach is its tendency to disregard conflict and play down the degree of independence that those inhabiting the role possess. There is also scope for exploitation within these roles as could be seen in the abuse of medical power and disempowerment of the patient or sick person (Sharp, 2010).

Application to practice

Consider the culture within the unit where you work. What are the shared values, beliefs and customs that you see being upheld within your day-to-day practice?

How might these influence your behaviour and relationships with colleagues and women and their families?

By way of contrast, **conflict theory** or **critical theory**, which has its origins in the work of Karl Marx (1818–1883) has its roots in the economic conflicts that exist between social classes within society. Whereas consensus theory emphasises the importance of having a **collective consciousness** to facilitate harmonious integration within society, conflict theorists emphasise social differences and disparities in wealth power and status that lead to conflicts between individuals and social groups (Browne, 2011). The German philosopher, economist and sociologist Karl Marx was another key figure within the development of sociological theory. He believed that the organisation of economic production is fundamental to the development of society. Marx believed that class conflict is inevitable in societies and his theory of social class is defined by the dominant idea of the conflicts between the **bourgeoisie** ruling classes and poorer working classes or **proletariat**.

Trigger

Maternal and infant mortality and perinatal reports have persistently shown a socioeconomic gradient with the highest rates of adverse perinatal outcomes and mortality occurring in the most socioeconomically disadvantaged groups (Hollowell et al., 2009; Department of Health, 2010). The Department of Health (DH) has commissioned a programme of work to strengthen the evidence base on interventions to reduce infant mortality, with a particular focus on reducing inequalities in infant mortality.

Consider the strategies that are in place within your unit to strengthen the delivery of maternity care to disadvantaged and vulnerable women. Do you think they are effective? For further information visit the National Perinatal Epidemiology Unit at: www.npeu.ox.ac.uk/infant-mortality

The focus of Marxism is based on capitalism, that is, an economic system based on the private ownership of the means of production and distribution of goods. Marx's writing chiefly focused on critiquing capitalism as a class structure that was characterised by division and exploitation and the overthrowing of capitalism by socialism. Communism was described as a theoretical ideal that would replace capitalism. There have been many attempts to apply Marxist theory to the study of health and a branch of Marxism termed neo-Marxism comprises of sociologists who have endeavoured to revise the original theories of Marx. The Frankfurt School, established in 1923, refers to a group of sociologists based at the Institute of Social Research in Frankfurt who sought to develop the work of Karl Marx to take into account the changes within society following his death.

The above sociological theories are characterised by their analysis of the way that society as a whole fits together, their focus being on structure as opposed to the individual or small groups. Such theories are referred to as structural theories or perspectives and are often described as **macro perspectives** because they focus on looking at the structure of whole societies and the implications of different ways of organising societies as opposed to the individual experience. Both functionalism and conflict theory are two main sociological theories that fall within the structural or macro perspective.

The interpretive approach and social action theories

Not all sociological perspectives base their approach upon the structure of society as a whole and instead consider the interaction between groups and individuals and stress the importance of the meaningfulness of human behaviour and interaction (Haralambos and Holborn, 2013), as opposed to the externalised structure of society. The German sociologist and political economist Max Weber (1864–1920) endeavoured to bridge the gulf between both macro and **micro approaches** to sociological theory while emphasising the importance of adopting a methodical, systematic and rigorous approach to sociological inquiry (Ritzer and Goodman, 2004).

Weber was influenced to some extent by Marx and viewed economic factors as being important when understanding the causes of social change, however he viewed class conflict as less significant than Marx (Giddens and Sutton, 2013) and emphasised that social change could come about in ways that did not just involve class conflicts. Instead Weber stressed the importance of *verstehen*, translated from German as meaning 'to understand', and sought to explain the meanings that individuals attribute to their interactions when considering causality (Ritzer and Goodman, 2004.)

An important part of Weber's sociological perspective was the proposal of the concept of an ideal type. An ideal type is an analytical construct that a sociologist may use as a benchmark or fixed point of reference (Giddens and Sutton, 2013) when establishing similarities as well as deviations in historical cases (Coser, 2003) and can help sociologists to explain and understand situations that occur within the world. An ideal type can be used to emphasise typical courses of conduct or social actions that might be expected for certain groups of people. Power was also an important concept to Weber and he made a significant contribution to the study of obedience and authority and distinguished three main modes of authority, each associated with its own forms of organisation and administration.

Trigger

Read the document *Implementing Human Factors in Healthcare*. Online at: www.patientsafetyfirst.nhs.uk/ashx/Asset.ashx?path=/Intervention-support/Human+Factors+How-to+Guide+v1.2.pdf

Consider case study one and the contributing factors that led to the woman's death. Think about the culture of your unit and whether you would feel able to raise any concerns aloud in the presence of senior clinicians. Does the hierarchy within your workplace make assertiveness difficult or do you work within a team where everyone has equal opportunity to have a voice? What potential impact might this have on the maintenance of a safe environment?

For Weber, therefore, society is created through social interaction that involves the conscious behaviour of rational, contemplative, individuals. For this reason Weber's approach is often referred to as a **social action theory** and is based upon an **interpretive** approach. Such an approach was largely developed to establish an alternative to the dominant positivist approach to sociology at the time when emphasis was placed on considering facts as they were observed objectively, without consideration being given to their underlying meaning (Bowling, 2009.) Thus an interpretative approach assumes that reality is not a fixed entity but exists within a context of which many constructions are possible (Polit and Beck, 2014).

It was around the same time that a group of American philosophers and sociologists from the University of Chicago who, building upon the work of Weber, developed a major theory of social action that became known as **symbolic interactionism** (Sharp, 2010). The American philosopher, sociologist and psychologist George Herbert Mead (1863–1931) was the most prominent figure in the development of this approach, although the term 'symbolic interactionism' was coined by a student of Mead's, Herbert Blumer (1900–1987).

Symbolic interactionism focuses on the detail of interpersonal interaction and how we can derive meaning from what others say and do from this (Giddens and Sutton, 2013). The use of language is a key concept for Mead, and indeed later symbolic interactionists, as he believed that the descriptive words that we use are in fact symbols that represent our meaning. It is through our shared understanding of symbols that humans are able to interact with each other. For Mead, both the mind and concept of self evolves or emerges as part of the process of socialisation (Mead, 1934) and so the self is socially rather than biologically constructed. It is through the use of shared symbols that language can be studied to explain the social reality.

Other branches of interpretive theory that have seen increasing popularity in recent times are **phenomenology** and **ethnomethodology**. Although the origins of phenomenological philosophy can be traced back hundreds of years, the Austrian philosopher and mathematician Edmund Husserl (1859–1938) is widely recognised as being the founder of the phenomenological movement (Morse and Richards, 2002; Patton, 2015; Robinson, 2006). Husserl was originally a mathematician whose interests in the problems of mathematics led him to logic and philosophy. Within his work he endeavoured to look beyond constructions, preconceptions and assumptions to the essence of the experience being studied. It was the Austrian social scientist Alfred Schutz (1899–1959) who, influenced by the work of both Husserl and Weber, developed phenomenology into a distinct sociological theory.

Schutz's phenomenological view emphasises that while our social life is a shared experience, it also ultimately anchored in the subjective experience of the individual subject (Overgaard and Zahavi, 2009). Thus Schutz moved attention away from the finding of meanings within a causal framework of social and historical conditions, as Weber had sought to do (David, 2010), and looked instead at how meaning can be derived from the individual experience.

The ethnomethodological approach was developed by the American sociologist Harold Garfinkel (1917–2011) with the intention of examining how human beings organise their social environment in a meaningful way. Like Schutz, the ethnomethodologist seeks to view things from the individual perspective and regards social structures such as groups and organisations as being the product of social interaction, rather than as pre-existing and determining factors. Social reality is thus conceived of as being a construction that is actively maintained by the participants (Overgaard and Zahavi, 2009.)

Other sociological theories

More recently attempts have been made to bridge the gap that existed between structural and interpretative theories. The British sociologist Anthony Giddens developed the theory **structuration** as a means of doing this and asserted that both structure and social action are closely related and that one cannot survive without the existence of the other. To illustrate this point Giddens (1984) has emphasised how both structure and social action function within a complementary role. Whereas structures enable social action to take place, social action helps to create structure. Giddens (1984) has used language as an example of structure and explains how while it is a necessary structure that enables people to communicate, it is the continual interaction and use of language by people over time that ensures the survival of language and indeed may contribute to the evolution of language and words.

Feminist theory as the name suggests is concerned with gender and seeks to address and explore inequalities of gender within society and places emphasis upon the experiences of women within society. It is beyond the scope of this chapter to do justice to the growing body of literature that emphasises the disadvantaged position of women in society, although the reader is directed to the following website for an overview of current inequalities that exist within the United Kingdom between men and women: www.fawcettsociety.org.uk.

Oakley (2005) suggested that the fundamental source of discrimination towards women can be found within social attitudes and beliefs and that this also pertains to the study of sociology, whereby greater prestige is assigned to traditionally male values and roles. This is also apparent when reading the findings of literature that has sought to explore midwives' roles within the workplace (see Table 1.1 and the research findings of Kirkham and Stapleton, 2000; and Rowan, 2003). There have been various discussions related to hierarchy and intimidation within midwifery literature (Curtis et al., 2006; Kirkham, 1999; Kirkham et al., 2006) and these will be explored in Chapter Two. However research that examines the social context within which predominantly female groups such as midwives work is crucial in helping to address the balance of power within clinical practice so that midwives feel able to support and empower the women in their care (Hunter and Warren, 2013; Kirkham, 1993).

Sociological research

Introduction to sociological research

This section provides an overview of the various approaches that are used by those engaged in research and to position social research within the context of sociology and describe its relevance to midwifery. An understanding and ability to evaluate relevant research forms a vital part of both pre- and post-registration midwifery curricula (NMC, 2009) and the Nursing and Midwifery Council (NMC) Code (NMC, 2015) clearly articulates that nurses, midwives and health visitors must use the best available evidence and keep their knowledge and skills updated. One of the strategic goals of the Royal College of Midwives (RCM) is to broaden and strengthen its research activities and national guidance has emphasised how maternity services should be measured in terms of actual and perceived safety, effectiveness of care and the experience of women and their partners (Department of Health, 2009; Midwifery 2020, 2010).

Methodologically sound research has explanatory and predictive powers and can be analysed in relation to other data to strengthen its findings. Having an understanding of research can empower midwives to better understand the experiences of the women and families that they care for. It also promotes **reflexivity** in so much as it shines a light on the experiences of midwives in practice and helps to empower midwives to challenge accepted practices, shape policy and guideline development and make positive changes for the benefits of the women in their care.

Sociological research has played a key part in the development of midwifery research and knowledge and proved valuable in examining the realities of midwifery practice and the experience of women and their families. Kingdon (2009) highlighted how the boundaries between sociological, midwifery and medical research have become increasingly hazy as midwives and other healthcare professionals increasingly scrutinise their practice through using a sociological perspective. Within their seminal work Hunt and Symonds (1995) undertook an ethnographic study of midwives at work within two British maternity units in order to explore the social meaning of midwifery and 'unravel their constructed occupational identity' (Hunt and Symonds, 1995, p. xv). There are many other varied examples of how sociological research has proved valuable in helping us to understand the culture within which we work as midwives and to challenge outdated practice. A few further examples are shown in Table 1.1 and the themes identified within these studies will be explored further in the following chapter where we consider the application of sociology to midwifery and the woman and her family.

Application to midwifery practice

Consider the research summarised in Table 1.1. How might these findings inform the way that you practice and your role within the multidisciplinary team? Consider other ways that sociological inquiry might influence the way that you practice.

Table 1.1 Examples of the use of sociological research within midwifery

Authors	Overview of study and research findings
Kirkham and Stapleton (2000)	Addressed midwives' support needs as they were described by midwives in England. Using a grounded theory approach for analysis, in-depth, ethnographic interviews were conducted with 168 midwives. The authors found that midwives lacked support, but interestingly did not see themselves as having parallel rights to this support when compared with the women they cared for. Respondents described the culture of midwifery within the NHS as a female culture of caring that was expressed through service and sacrifice that operated within institutions that did not value the importance of such caring work. Kirkham and Stapleton (2000) suggest that this reflected a culture of midwifery that held deeply ingrained values of service and self-sacrifice.
Green and Baird (2009)	Undertook an exploratory study to investigate students' experiences that lead to both attrition and retention. The authors found a perceived lack of support within clinical practice, the emotional demands of midwifery and balancing the demands of theory and practice were among the main emerging themes. Students from the three-year direct-entry programme spent a long time trying to 'fit in' (Green and Baird, 2009, p.6) with clinical practice as they had not had the degree of socialisation that the 78-week midwifery students had because of their previous nurse training.
Rowan (2003)	Undertook a phenomenological study to gain an in-depth understanding of what it is like to be a midwife without children. Nearly all midwives within her study were asked by the women they cared for whether they had children and Rowan (2003) concluded that the midwives' views reflected the expectation within society that most women would become mothers. Whereas some of the midwives within her study felt that not having children made them more objective in giving care, some also felt a degree of inadequacy because they did not have children.

Authors	Overview of study and research findings
de Jonge et al. (2004)	Undertook a meta-analysis study in order to establish whether the continuation of the routine use of the supine position during labour was justified. The findings revealed that there were a higher rate of instrumental deliveries and episiotomies in the supine position although a lower estimated blood loss and lower rate of postpartum haemorrhage were found in the supine position. Many methodological problems were identified within the included studies by de Jong et al. (2004) and the appropriateness of a randomised controlled trial to study this subject was questioned. The authors recommended instead that a cohort study would be a more appropriate methodology, supplemented by a qualitative method to study women's experiences. In addition de Jong et al. (2004) emphasised the importance of using objective laboratory measurements when examining the difference in blood loss rather than observation, which is subject to differences in interpretation and as such a possible source of bias. De Jong et al. (2004) concluded that the results from the meta-analysis did not justify the continuation of the routine use of the supine position during the second stage of labour.

Closely linked with sociological theory, sociological research seeks to evaluate outcomes, explain problems, behaviour and experiences and inform us about the culture within which we work as shown within the examples provided within Table 1.1. The study of sociology involves confronting a wide range of ethical issues and, in particular, sociological research has been influential in identifying inequalities in health and the experiences of women and their families and midwives working within the maternity setting.

Theoretical frameworks and assumptions underpinning sociological research

Like sociological theories themselves, methods of social research are closely tied to different perspectives and theories of how social reality should be studied. As we have seen in the previous section, many different viewpoints and theories regarding the nature of society and the social world have been proposed and it is important to remember that within sociological research the **research methods** used to carry out the research should be aligned with both the research **methodology** and the theoretical assumptions of the researcher regarding the nature of the reality being studied.

This theoretical framework is sometimes referred to as the **paradigm** or worldview, within which the research methodology sits (Bowling, 2009) and guides the way that knowledge is then generated and interpreted. It is the choice of paradigm that sets down the intent, stimulus and expectations for the research as without this there is no basis for subsequent choices regarding methodology, methods, literature or research design (Mackenzie and Knipe, 2006). Many research textbooks also refer to **epistemology** when discussing the world view within which the research sits and Crotty (1998) defined this as the theory of knowledge, which is embedded within the research methodology itself and which demonstrates the relationship between the researcher to the research (Bryman, 2012).

It is also important to note the distinction between research methodology and research methods as this is not always clearly defined within research textbooks. Silverman (2006) defined these concepts very simply by stating that the research methodology describes the researcher's general approach to the research and defines how the researcher will go about studying a phenomenon and the research methods as the specific techniques used for carrying out the research. Within sociological research it is important that the research methods used align with the chosen research methodology that should also align with the theoretical perspective within which the generation of knowledge will sit.

There are many research books that provide a comprehensive and thorough overview of the main assumptions that dominate our worldview and the associated appropriate research methodologies and methods, for example Bryman (2012) and Patton (2015). Having an understanding of the theoretical assumptions within which a particular research theory sits is important to help us to understand the context for the research findings. Polit and Beck (2014) have also emphasised, however, that all researchers share common goals and are faced with similar challenges and constraints despite their individual philosophic and methodological differences.

The scientific approach and overview of quantitative research methods

The traditional scientific approach that has dominated research has its roots in the philosophical paradigm positivism. As previously discussed this was prominent in the theory of the early nineteenth-century philosophers and sociologists such as Comte and Durkheim. The fundamental assumption of those that subscribe to a positivist approach is that there is an external objective world reality that can be studied according to the principles of the **scientific method** and to which the researcher is independent.

In order to further describe the link between theories and research it is important to consider the research question itself and whether data are collected to test or build theories (Bryman, 2012). **Deductive** reasoning is used within the positivist approach to research whereby findings are generated from an initial theory that is developed into a testable hypothesis that can then be rigorously tested in order to be accepted or rejected. Within the scientific approach it is important that the proposed hypothesis is **operationally defined,** that is, it is translated in such a way that the researcher is able to clearly articulate the systematic process and research methods used in order to determine whether the initial theory or hypothesis can be accepted or rejected.

Deductive theory is rooted in **empiricism**. Empiricism is a term used to suggest that only evidence gained through the external senses that is rooted in an objective reality is acceptable and ideas must be scrutinised through rigorous testing before they can be considered knowledgeable. Mechanisms are therefore put in place to **control** the research study so that any possible **biases** are eliminated or reduced as much as possible so that the **internal and external validity** of the study is enhanced. Another important aim of the scientific approach is to state the degree to which the findings of the study can be **generalised** to other individuals.

The scientific approach is commonly associated with **quantitative research** (Bryman, 2012) and the most popular quantitative research methods that are used within healthcare include randomised controlled trials (RCT), cohort studies, longitudinal studies, other experimental methods and surveys, all of which produce numerical data requiring data analysis using statistical techniques. An overview of some of the main quantitative research methods is provided in Table 1.2.

The scientific approach has enjoyed considerable stature as a method of inquiry (Polit and Beck, 2004) and Cluett (2006) acknowledged that not all types of research are valued to the same degree. Evidence-based practice has evolved from the term evidence-based medicine which Sackett et al. (1996) defined as the conscientious, explicit and judicious use of current best evidence in making decisions about the care of individual patients. This is evident in the allocation of resources and publication and dissemination of findings from published trials within healthcare.

Guyatt et al.'s (1995) hierarchy of research locates systematic reviews and meta-analyses at the top of the hierarchy followed by randomised controlled trials. The Cochrane database has been at the forefront of systematic review methodology for over two decades and Walsh (2007) has suggested that maternity services were pioneers within the birth of the evidence-based practice culture due to the formulation of the Cochrane database. Cochrane systematic reviews seek to collate all evidence that fits prespecified eligibility criteria in order to address a specific research question

Table 1.2 An overview of quantitative research methods

Paradigm theoretical perspective	Quantitative research methods	Data collection tools	Data analysis
Scientific approach Positivist	Experimental designs, e.g. randomised controlled trials, factorial designs	Biophysical measurements	Data coding and assignment of numerical values
	Non-experimental designs e.g. correlational designs and case control designs	Structured questionnaires Structured interviews	Data entry and appropriate statistical analysis depending on type of numerical data generated
	Survey or cross-sectional designs, evaluation research, meta-analysis	Structured observation	

(Higgins and Green, 2011). The database has a strict inclusion criterion that uses explicit systematic methods to minimise bias and increase the reliability of the findings and conclusions drawn from these (Higgins and Green, 2011).

Criticisms of the scientific approach include the issue that by its very nature it is **reductionist** that is it reduces the human experience to only the few concepts under investigation that are predetermined by the investigator (Polit and Beck, 2004). For this reason it has been viewed as misleading as it stresses the significance of external facts without understanding the underlying mechanisms observed or their meaning to individuals (Bowling, 2009.) Indeed, Schutz (1970) suggested that positivism misses the progress that is to be made in the objective exploration of the human subjective experience.

Sandall and McCandlish (2006) argued that rather than accepting hierarchies of evidence we should consider what really matters, that is ensuring that the research method is chosen to fit the research question. The acceptance that knowledge generation is significant only when it is able to establish causal relationships and correlations between identified variables seems limited. It is more appropriate therefore to herald this approach as the 'gold standard' of research methods only when the question to be answered is one of effectiveness or outcomes (Sandall and McCandlish, 2006; Sakala and Corry, 2001).

The interpretative approach and qualitative research methods

The **interpretative approach** began as a counter movement to positivism and the scientific method and incorporates different branches of theory and research methodology that include social action theory, symbolic interactionism, ethnomethodology and phenomenology. Often referred to as **constructivism** it is underpinned by the belief that knowledge and human understanding of the world is constructed by us and through our interpretations of the real world (Kingdon, 2009).

Research that utilises an interpretative approach uses **inductive reasoning**, whereby theory is generated from observations and findings. Such an approach is associated with the use of **qualitative research** and Table 1.3 provides an overview of some of the main qualitative research methods.

Table 1.3 An overview of qualitative research methods

Paradigm and theoretical perspective	Qualitative research methods	Data collection tools	Data analysis
Interpretative or constructionist	Ethnography Phenomenology Grounded theory Case studies	Participant observation Unstructured/ semi-structured interviews Focus groups Document or text analysis	Reading the data Assignment of codes Assignment of categories Developing analytical constructs Interpreting the data

Table 1.4 Main differences between qualitative and quantitative research

Quantitative	Qualitative
Numbers – statistical analysis	Words
Researcher perspective	Permits participant perspectives
Search for causal relationship	Incorporate researcher reflexivity
Theory driven	Theory emerges from the data
Structured	Unstructured
Generalisable	Contextual understanding
Hard reliable data	Rich, deep data
Macro perspective	Micro perspective
Objective behaviour	Meaning
Artificial controlled settings	Naturalistic settings

Source: Adapted from Bryman, 2004, p. 287

More recently the use of qualitative research methods, notably phenomenology, has gained popularity within healthcare as their potential value has been recognised (Department of Health, 2007). Phenomenology is concerned with understanding the lived experiences of individuals (Byrne, 2001) and believes that these experiences give meaning to each person's perception of individual phenomena (Polit and Beck, 2004). Common to all interpretive research is the focus on exploring how as humans we make sense of our experiences (Patton, 2015) and Table 1.4 demonstrates the main differences between qualitative and quantitative research.

However the proliferation of such interpretive research and particularly phenomenology within nursing, midwifery and healthcare settings has not been without strong criticism (Crotty, 1996, 1998; Paley, 1997). This may in part be due to the various approaches that have evolved under the umbrella of phenomenology and other qualitative research methods that have resulted in a lack of uniformity in the concepts and language used to describe its research methods and methodology.

Whereas the notion of the researcher is removed from quantitative research methods, qualitative research methods generally acknowledge the presence of and potential influence of the researcher upon the data collected. The concept of **reflexivity** within qualitative research and in particular ethnography and phenomenology emphasises the need to make transparent and overt the researcher's own personal values, background and cultural suppositions (Gearing, 2004). By being transparent about the researcher's own personal values, background and cultural suppositions it is hoped that their possible impact on the phenomena under investigation will be minimised and at least provide the reader with enough information to assess for themselves the trustworthiness and credibility of the research findings.

Unlike quantitative research, there is increased scope for flexibility within qualitative research designs where the emergent theory may lead the researcher to explore new avenues of inquiry. This does not mean, however, that the researcher adopts a less rigorous approach when considering issues relating to validity and **reliability**. LeCompte and Goetz (1982) emphasised that a concern with validity and reliability should be

Table 1.5 Lincoln and Guba's translation of terms for establishing rigour in interpretative inquiry

Scientific approach	Interpretative approach
Internal validity	Credibility
External validity	Transferability
Reliability	Dependability
Objectivity	Confirmability

Source: Cited in Seale, 1999, p. 45

shared by all social researchers; however it is important to note that the specific techniques for establishing validity and reliability must differ according to the research methodology.

It has been suggested that while the terms reliability and validity are appropriate for research that adopts a scientific approach, such terms are inappropriate for qualitative enquiry (Koch and Harrington, 1998). Lincoln and Guba (1985) sought to translate the terms used within the scientific method so that they are appropriate for interpretative approaches to research (see Table 1.5). Robson (2002) suggested that the problem lies in the fact that these terms have historically been operationalised rigidly within quantitative research. It is therefore important to try and find alternative ways of operationalising them that are appropriate to the conditions and circumstances of a qualitative research design. Seale (1999) used Lincoln and Guba's (1985) translation of terms to demonstrate an appropriate way for establishing rigour within interpretative inquiry in comparison to scientific inquiry. This has been adapted within Table 1.5 to demonstrate how rigour can be successfully articulated within both the scientific and interpretative approach to research.

Conclusion

This chapter has introduced the reader to some of the main sociological theories and research methods used within sociological inquiry. It has also endeavoured to consider how some of the key sociological concepts can be applied within midwifery practice and encouraged the reader to think critically about their own perspectives and the culture within which they work. As previously emphasised, the role of sociological inquiry is recognised as being crucial to examining the context within which we operate and shining a lens on our own perceptions and experiences. The next chapter considers in more detail the broader political, cultural, social and economic factors that impact upon our role, professional responsibilities and the women and families that we care for.

References

Bowling, A. (2009) *Research Methods in Health – Investigating Health and Health Services.* Third Edition. Maidenhead: Open University Press

British Sociological Association (n.d.) What is sociology? Available: http://www.britsoc. co.uk/WhatIsSociology/SocHist.aspx Accessed 1 September 2013

Browne, K. (2011) *An Introduction to Sociology.* Fourth Edition. Cambridge: Polity Press

Bryman, A. (2004) *Social Research Methods.* Second Edition. Oxford: Oxford University Press

Bryman, A. (2012) *Social Research Methods.* Fourth Edition. Oxford: Oxford University Press

Byrne, M. (2001) Understanding life experiences through a phenomenological approach to research. *AORN Journal* Volume 73, Issue 4, pp. 830–32

Cluett, E. R. (2006) Evidence based practice. In Cluett, E.R. and Bluff, R. (eds) *Principles and Practice of Research in Midwifery.* Second Edition. Edinburgh: Churchill Livingstone, pp. 33–53

Comte, A. (1854) *A General View of Positivism.* Translated from the French of Auguste Comte by J.H. Bridges M.B. Available online: https://archive.org/stream/ageneralview ofpo00comtuoft#page/n3/mode/thumb Accessed 1 July 2014

Coser, L. A. (2003) *Masters of Sociological Thought: Ideas in Historical and Social Context.* Second Edition. Illinois: Waveland Press Inc.

Crotty, M. (1996) *Phenomenology and Nursing Research.* London: Churchill Livingstone

Crotty, M. (1998) *The Foundations of Social Research: Meaning and Perspective in the Research Process.* London: Sage Publications

Curtis, P., Ball, L. and Kirkham, M. (2006) Bullying and horizontal violence: cultural or individual phenomena? *British Journal of Midwifery* Volume 14, No. 4, pp. 218–221

David, M. (2010) *Methods of Interpretive Sociology.* (SAGE Benchmarks in Social Research Methods). Thousand Oaks, California: SAGE Publications Ltd

De Jonge, A., Teunissen, T. A. M., Lagro-Janssen and A. L. M. (2004) Supine position compared to other positions during the second stage of labor: a meta-analytic review *Journal of Psychosomatic Obstetrics & Gynecology* Volume 25, Issue 1 , pp. 35–45

Department of Health *(2007) Maternity Matters.* London: Crown Copyright

Department of Health (2009) *Delivering High Quality Midwifery Care: The priorities, opportunities and challenges for midwives.* London: Crown Copyright

Department of Health (2010) *Tackling Health Inequalities in Infant and Maternal Health Outcomes. Report of the Infant Mortality National Support Team.* London: Crown Copyright

Gearing, R. E. (2004) Bracketing in research: A typology. *Qualitative Health Research* Volume 14, No.10, pp. 1429–1452

Giddens, A. (1984) *The Constitution of Society.* Cambridge: Polity Press

Giddens, A. and Sutton, P.W. (2013) *Sociology.* Seventh Edition. Cambridge: Polity Press

Green, S. and Baird, K. (2009) An exploratory, comparative study investigating attrition and retention of student midwives. *Midwifery* Volume 25, No. 1, pp. 79–87

Guyatt, G. H., Sackett, D. L., Sinclair, J. C., Hayward, R., Cook, D. J. and Cook, R. J. (1995) Users' guides to the medical literature. IX. A method for grading health care recommendations. *JAMA* Volume 274, pp.1800–04.

Haralambos, M. and Holborn, M. (2004) *Sociology Themes and Perspectives.* Sixth Edition. London: Collins

Haralambos, M. and Holborn, M. (2013) *Sociology Themes and Perspectives.* Eighth Edition. London: Collins

Higgins, J.P.T. and Green, S. (eds) (2011) *Cochrane Handbook for Systematic Reviews of Interventions.* Version 5.1.0 [updated March 2011]. The Cochrane Collaboration, 2011. Available from www.cochrane-handbook.org Accessed 14 November 2014

Hollowell, J., Kurinczuk, J., Oakley, L., Brocklehurst, P. and Gray, R. (2009) *A Systematic Review of the Effectiveness of Antenatal Care Programmes to Reduce Infant Mortality and its Major Causes in Socially Disadvantaged and Vulnerable Women – Final Report.* University of Oxford: National Perinatal Epidemiology Unit. Available: https://www. npeu.ox.ac.uk/downloads/files/infant-mortality/Infant-Mortality-Antenatal-Care-Report.pdf Accessed 4 July 2014

Hunt, S. and Symonds, A. (1995) *The Social Meaning of Midwifery.* London: Macmillan

Hunter, B. and Warren, L. (2013) *Investigating Resilience in Midwifery: Final Report.* Cardiff University: Cardiff

Kingdon, C. (2009) *Sociology for Midwives.* London: Quay Books MA Healthcare Ltd.

Kirkham, M. (1993) *Communication in Midwifery.* In: Alexander, J., Levy, V. and Roch, S. (eds) *Midwifery Practice-A Research Based Approach.* London: Macmillan Press, Chapter One.

Kirkham, M. (1999) The culture of midwifery in the NHS in England. *Journal of Advanced Nursing* Volume 30, No. 3, pp. 732–39

Kirkham, M. and Stapleton, H. (2000) Midwives support needs as childbirth changes. *Journal of Advanced Nursing* Volume 32, No. 2, pp. 465–72

Kirkham, M., Morgan, R. and Davies, C. (2006) *Why Do Midwives Stay?* London: Royal College of Midwives.

Koch, T. and Harrington, A. (1998) Reconceptualising rigour: The case for reflexivity. *Journal of Advanced Nursing* Volume 28, No. 4, pp. 882–90

LeCompte, M. and Goetz, J. (1982) Problems of reliability and validity in ethnographic research. *Review of Educational Research* Volume 52, No. 1, pp. 31–60

Lincoln, Y. S. and Guba, E. G. (1985) *Naturalistic Enquiry.* Newbury Park, California: Sage Publications

Mackenzie, N. and Knipe, S. (2006) Research dilemmas: Paradigms, methods and methodology. *Educational Research* Volume 16, No. 2, pp. 193–205. *Available:* http://www.iier.org.au/iier16/mackenzie.htmlVol 16 Accessed 23 July 2014

Mead, G. H. (1934) *Mind, Self, and Society.* Chicago: University of Chicago Press

Midwifery 2020 (2010) *Delivering Expectations.* Midwifery 2020 Programme. Available: http://midwifery2020.org.uk/documents/M2020Deliveringexpectations-FullReport2.pdf Accessed 1 November 2014

Morse, J. M. and Richards, L. (2002) *Read Me First for a Users Guide to Qualitative Methods.* Thousand Oaks, California: Sage Publications

NMC (National Midwifery Council) (2009*) Standards for Pre-registration Midwifery Education.* London: NMC

NMC (2015) *The Code. Professional Standards of Practice and Behaviour for Nurses and Midwives.* London: NMC. Available: http://www.nmc-uk.org/Documents/NMC-Publications/NMC-Code-A5-FINAL.pdf last accessed February 2015

Oakley, A. (2005) *The Ann Oakley Reader: Gender, women and social science.* Bristol: The Policy Press

Overgaard, S. and Zahavi, D. (2009) *Phenomenological Sociology: The subjectivity of everyday life.* In Jacobsen, M. H. (ed.) *Encountering the Everyday: An Introduction to the Sociologies of the Unnoticed.* Basingstoke: Palgrave Macmillan, pp. 93–115

Paley, J. (1997) Husserl, phenomenology and nursing. *Journal of Advanced Nursing* Volume 26, pp. 187–93

Patton, M. Q. (2015) *Qualitative Research and Evaluation Methods: Integrating Theory and Practice.* Fourth Edition. Thousand Oaks, California: Sage Publications

Polit, D. F and Beck, C. T. (2004) *Nursing Research: Principles and Methods.* Seventh Edition. Philadelphia: Lippincott Williams & Wilkins

Polit, D. F. and Beck, C. T. (2014) *Essentials of Nursing Research: Appraising Evidence for Nursing Practice.* Eighth Edition. Philadelphia: Wolters Kluwer: Lippincott Williams & Wilkins

Ritzer, G. and Goodman, D. (2004) *Modern Sociological Theory*. Sixth Edition. New York: McGraw Hill Companies

Robinson, A. (2006) Phenomenology. In Cluett, E. and Bluff, R. (eds) *Principles and Practice of Research in Midwifery*. Second Edition. Edinburgh: Churchill Livingstone, pp. 187–200

Robson, C. (2002) *Real World Research*. Second Edition. Oxford: Blackwell Publishing

Rowan, C. (2003) Midwives without children. *British Journal of Midwifery* Volume 11, No. 11, pp. 28–33

Sackett, D., Rosenburg, W., Gray, J., Haynes, B. and Richardson, W.S. (1996) Evidence based medicine: What it is and what it isn't. *British Medical Journal* Volume 312, pp. 71–72

Sakala, C. and and Corry, M. P. (2001) What is evidence based health care? *Journal of Midwifery and Woman's Health* Volume 46, No. 3, pp. 127–28

Sandall, J. and McCandlish, R. (2006) Why do research? In Page, L. and McCandlish, R. (eds) *The New Midwifery. Science and Sensitivity in Practice*. Second Edition. London: Churchill Livingstone, pp. 251–71

Schutz, A. (1970) Concept and theory formation in the social sciences. In: Emmet, D. and MacIntyre, A. (eds) *Sociological Theory and Philosophical Analysis*. London: Macmillan, pp. 1–19

Seale, C. (1999) *The Quality of Qualitative Research*. London: Sage publications

Sharp, K. (2010) What is sociology? In Denny, E. and Earle, S. (eds) *Sociology for Nurses*. Second Edition. Cambridge: Polity Press, pp.7–28

Silverman, D. (2006) *Interpreting Qualitative Data*. Third Edition. Los Angeles: Sage Publications

Walsh, D. (2007) *Evidence Based Care for Normal Labour and Birth*. London: Routledge

2 Application of sociology to midwifery

Kate Nash

Aim

The aim of this chapter is to offer an overview of the broader political, cultural and social factors that impact upon the role of the midwife, our professional responsibilities and the women and families that we care for. Through reading this chapter the reader will critically consider how midwives can successfully negotiate these factors in order to facilitate the formation of positive working relationships and overcome the challenges that may be presented along the way.

Learning outcomes

By the end of this chapter the reader will be able to:

- Consider the history of midwifery within the United Kingdom and how it has shaped our role within society today
- Recognise the impact that the organisation of maternity services and regulation of midwifery has upon midwifery care today
- Critically reflect upon the role of the midwife within the broader sociological climate and culture within which midwifery care is delivered
- Explore the broader sociological factors that impact upon the childbearing woman and her family
- Understand the sociological factors that might influence the relationships that midwives form with their colleagues, women and their families
- Discuss how midwives might negotiate any challenges that they face within today's society to provide optimal care for childbearing women and their families

---

Introduction

Relationships form the bedrock of midwifery practice and midwives must strive to develop and sustain meaningful relationships with women and their families, the wider multi-professional team and society as a whole. By examining society on both a macro and micro perspective, lessons can be learned about the organisational climate and culture within which we work. This will ultimately enable us to reflect upon both individual practice and maternity care as a whole to strive to improve the working climate for midwives and care that is provided for women and their families.

This chapter is divided into two sections. Section one considers the history and regulation of midwifery and the organisational factors that impact upon maternity services. The midwife's role will be viewed within both a historical and current day context and consideration given to how a positive working culture can be established to facilitate the promotion of professional relations and women-centred care. Section two focuses on the childbearing woman and her family. The impact of issues such as changing population demographics, social media and expectations regarding the delivery of maternity social inequalities will be explored.

The history and regulation of midwifery – an overview of the organisational factors that impact upon maternity services

The history of midwifery has been discussed in much detail by many authors (Donnison, 1988; Leap and Hunter, 1993; Towler and Bramall, 1986) and there are varying historical accounts of midwifery practice. Midwives are mentioned throughout history and can be traced back to biblical times, however their path to professional status has been extensive and troubled (Symonds and Hunt, 1996), with many sources detailing the inconsistency in standards of practice among midwives and the negative image often ascribed to midwifery because of adverse publicity that emphasised the dangers of incompetent practitioners (Borrelli, 2013; Tew, 1998).

Borrelli (2013) suggests that the first textbook of midwifery was written by the physician Soranus of Ephesus during the second century AD, and proceeds to describe the prerequisite characteristics of midwives during the sixteenth, seventeenth and eighteenth centuries as defined by physicians at that time. These tended to focus on the perceived value of midwives' various physical and personality attributes. Within the nineteenth century an examination for midwives was introduced by the London Obstetrical Society (founded in 1858) with the intention of improving midwives' professional status, although the resulting diploma was not officially or legally recognised (Mayes, 1930).

The Trained Midwives' Registration Society was formed in 1881 in an attempt to improve the status and competence of midwives and was founded by Zepherina Veitch, a midwife who worked with the poor at the British Lying-In Hospital in London, and Louisa Hubbard, the editor of a women's journal called *Work and Leisure* (RCM, n.d.) The name of the society was changed to the Midwives Institute in 1886 and evolved to become the Royal College of Midwives (RCM) in 1941 although its

Royal Charter was received in 1947. The society was pivotal in improving the standing of midwives within society through better education and recommendations that the profession of midwifery be set in statute. However it was not until 1902 when the Central Midwives Board was set up by the Midwives Act (1902) (Parliament, 1902) that legislation was passed to assure improved training, regulation and control for midwifery practice. This prevented unqualified and unregistered women from practicing midwifery and only those midwives certified under the act were able to practice as midwives within England and Wales. This consisted of women who already possessed a recognised qualification in midwifery in addition to those women considered to be of good character who had at least one year's prior experience of attending women in childbirth (Nuttall, 2012).

The resulting legislation cited several rules and features that were considered essential for safe midwifery practice and was crucial in securing the future for the profession of midwifery. This was because it provided an established system of recognition and registration for midwives and marked an end to the general perception of midwives as being of an inferior social status and professional position (Royal College of Obstetricians and Gynaecologists, 2012). It is evident that at this time there was a clear need for midwifery practice to be strengthened by a sound physiological knowledge base, development of professional skills and the integration of psychosocial care with scientific knowledge and this view was supported by the earlier writings of Florence Nightingale (Nightingale, 1871).

During the early-twentieth century the usual place for women to birth their babies was at home (Dodwell and Newburn, 2010); however by the 1930s, the two leading models of care were a consultant-based hospital system and a community-based maternal and child health system. The move to a state-remunerated midwifery service was completed in 1936 with the passing of the 1936 Midwives Act, which was seen as part of the solution to the high levels of maternal mortality that existed at the time (Benoit et al., 2005). The goal was to provide a national salaried community-based midwifery service, including antenatal and postnatal care, home birth and general practitioner (GP) back up. Between the late-1940s and mid-1960s approximately two-thirds of births in England and Wales took place in hospital and one-third at home. The move away from home births took place largely between 1963 and 1974, during which time the percentage of women giving birth at home fell from 30 per cent to 4.2 per cent (ONS, 2012). Instrumental in this shift from home to hospital birth was the creation of the National Health Service (NHS) in 1948, which generated renewed interest in maternal health (Davis, 2013) and provided women with the right to free maternity care while reinforcing the role of medically led hospital services.

The Maternity and Midwifery Advisory Committee was asked to consider the future of maternity services in 1967 and the subsequent Peel report, named after the committee chair, Consultant Obstetrician John Peel, recommended that all births take place in hospital with medical and midwifery care provided by consultant obstetricians, GPs and midwives working as teams (Standing Maternity and Midwifery Advisory Committee, 1970). Therefore although midwives continued to be the main attendant at hospital births, their role became disjointed largely as a result of increasing medical dominance (Benoit et al., 2005) and precedence given to the assumed authoritative knowledge of doctors, based on scientific principles, and perceived safety of consultant-led hospital birth. See Box 2.1 for a definition of authoritative knowledge

---

Box 2.1 Definition of authoritative knowledge

Authoritative knowledge has been defined by Davis-Floyd and Sargeant (1997) as the specialised knowledge that a professional holds that provides the foundation for status and social distance between the 'expert' and the woman, as the woman is deemed to be barred from the impenetrable knowledge of the professional.

The use of scientific and technological expertise through the **medicalisation** of birth within a hospital setting was deemed fundamental in improving the safety for women and babies. Much criticism existed regarding the recommendations of the Peel report and its subsequent impact upon maternity care and it was emphasised that such recommendations failed to seek the views of the users of maternity services or indeed were based on any robust supporting evidence. Marjorie Tew, a statistician who taught medical students how they could use statistics to gather information about diseases, found that the relevant routine birth statistics collected 'failed to support the widely accepted hypothesis that the increased hospitalization of birth had caused the decline achieved in the mortality of mothers and newborn babies' (Tew, 1998, p. viii). She faced enormous resistance to her findings from the medical community who initially refused to discuss her criticisms of their established practice or publish her findings (Tew, 1985). Thus the move to hospital birth can be viewed as one of the greatest sociological changes within the latter part of the twentieth century, despite the fact that there was no robust evidence to support this change at the time.

Application to practice

Recently the National Perinatal Epidemiology Unit (established in 1978) published their findings from the birthplace study (Birthplace in England Collaborative Group, 2011). These are large prospective cohort studies that aim to compare perinatal outcomes, maternal outcomes and interventions in labour by planned place of birth at the start of care in labour for women with low-risk pregnancies. The sample size consisted of 64,538 eligible women with a singleton, term and 'booked' pregnancy who gave birth between April 2008 and April 2010 in England. The results showed that women planning birth in a midwifery unit and multiparous women planning birth at home experience fewer interventions than those planning birth in an obstetric unit with no impact on perinatal outcomes. For nulliparous women, planned home births also have fewer interventions but have poorer perinatal outcomes and a higher transfer rate from non-obstetric settings. The authors concluded that the results support a policy of offering healthy women with low-risk pregnancies a choice of birth setting. For further details visit: https://www.npeu.ox.ac.uk/birthplace.

Currently the homebirth rate remains low at about 2.3 per cent (ONS, 2012). Consider how women's choice with regards to their place of birth is supported at your unit. What tools are in place to facilitate choice (e.g. leaflets, provision of information) and are there any factors that might inhibit women's choice?

The publication and recommendations of the Briggs report in 1972 (DHSS, 1972) led to the review of the role and training of both nurses and midwives and recommended a united statutory structure for nurses, midwives and health visitors. These recommendations formed the basis for the Nurses, Midwives and Health Visitors Act in 1979 (Parliament, 1979) and the establishment of the United Kingdom Central Council for Nursing, Midwifery and Health Visiting (UKCC) and the four national boards in 1983. These changes were not welcomed by all midwives who felt that the role and status of the midwife as an independent practitioner was in danger of becoming blurred with nursing and argued for amendments to the legislation to be made to ensure that the voice of midwifery was strengthened (Royal College of Obstetricians and Gynaecologists Heritage Collections Blog, 2013). Such arguments were also supported by the obstetrician and secretary general of the International Federation of Gynaecology and Obstetrics (FIGO), John Tomkinson, who was nominated by the Royal College of Obstetricians and Gynaecologists (RCOG) as a point of contact in governmental debates. Tomkinson strongly emphasised the full support that the RCOG gave to the professional status of midwifery (Royal College of Obstetricians and Gynaecologists Heritage Collections Blog, 2013). A summary of the functions of the previous UKCC and the Nursing Midwifery Council (NMC) is highlighted in Box 2.2.

Box 2.2   Summary of the functions of the UKCC and NMC

The main purpose of the UKCC was to maintain a register of UK nurses, midwives and health visitors, provide guidance to registrants and handle professional misconduct complaints (Nursing Midwifery Council, 2010). This arrangement continued with minor alterations up to April 2002, when the UKCC and national boards came to an end and its functions were taken over by a new Nursing and Midwifery Council. The NMC is currently the statutory regulator of nurses and midwives in the UK and is required by the Nursing and Midwifery Order in 2001 (Stationery Office, 2002) to establish and maintain a register of all qualified nurses and midwives eligible to practise in the UK, to set standards for their education, practice and conduct, and to take action when those standards are called into question. The NMC also has the power to set rules for the regulation of the practice of midwives (NMC, 2012).

As the medical dominance of birth continued, the value of midwifery-led care and views of women appeared diminished, although a backlash existed among some midwives and consumer-led groups. Prunella Briance, who had herself suffered from traumatic experiences while giving birth, launched the Natural Childbirth Association of Great Britain in 1957. This later became a charitable trust and changed its name to the National Childbirth Trust (NCT). The organisation was established to promote natural childbirth and ensure all parents-to-be and new parents had a voice and felt supported, informed and confident regarding matters pertaining to childbirth.

It was also around this time that another voluntary organisation, the Society for the Prevention of Cruelty to Pregnant Women, renamed in 1960 to the Association for Improvements in the Maternity Services (AIMS), was founded by Sally Willington following her distressing antenatal and birth experience with the aim of campaigning for improved NHS care for parents and an end to the routine use of degrading measures employed routinely during childbirth. These included pubic shaves, enemas to open the bowels prior to childbirth and episiotomies (AIMS, 2010). AIMS has since worked closely with another charity the Association of Radical Midwives (ARM), set up in 1976 to improve the maternity care provided by the NHS. These groups have gained momentum over time and proved to be pivotal in shaping government policy and raising the importance of maternal rights and the importance of individual care with a focus on control, choice and respect for dignity.

Fortunately the 1980s saw the introduction of **evidence-based practice** and research began to play a crucial part in legitimising the concerns expressed by the consumer-led groups (Benoit et al., 2005). The publication of *Effective Care in Pregnancy and Childbirth* (Chalmers et al., 1989) provided an overview of the best evidence available to inform and underpin clinical practice and it became clear that many obstetric-led practices such as episiotomy (Graham, 1997) and electronic fetal monitoring (Graham et al., 2004) had been implemented prior to sufficient evaluation (Sakala and Corry, 2008).

The involvement of women who used maternity services within service planning and strategy was further increased by the development of **Maternity Service Liaison Committees** (MSLCs) within England in 1984. These aimed to provide local forums where women who had used maternity services could plan how best to meet the needs of the local population of childbearing women. However it was important that such forums became more than just a government tick box exercise and their role has more recently been strengthened by statute through the implementation of several key government documents (Department of Health, 1993, 2007) and national guidelines that emphasise the importance of MSLCs having a multidisciplinary function (Department of Health, 2006a).

Although technological intervention within childbirth continued to grow through-out the 1980s, these organisations played a vital role in publicising debates within childbirth leading to both governmental and media attention. An Expert Maternity Group chaired by Baroness Cumberlege, then parliamentary under-secretary of state at the Department of Health, undertook a review of maternity services which made rec-ommendations for improvement through the publication of *Changing Childbirth* (Department of Health, 1993). Integral to the key principles of the report was the desire to finally make women the focus of their own maternity care so that women felt in control of what was happening, had choice and were able to make decisions about their own care based on their individual needs, having discussed matters with the health professionals involved with their care.

The publication and implementation of this report appeared to have little impact within the reality of clinical practice and qualitative research undertaken to explore women's views about their childbirth experiences demonstrated that issues relating to choice, control and support for women continued to be an important issue that needed addressing (Berg et al., 1996; Berg and Dahlberg, 1998; Green et al., 2003; Green and Baston, 2003; Hall and Holloway, 1998; Hodnett et al., 2007). More recently the publication of *Maternity Matters* (Department of Health, 2007) reemphasised the themes outlined within *Changing Childbirth* and reiterated the government's commitment to offering control, choice and continuity of care by the end of 2009. Fundamental to this was for women to be offered a choice with regards to the type of care that they received, pain relief available to them and place of birth, and these principles continue to have been adopted by the current Coalition government.

Thus we can see how historically both midwives and women have been perceived to be subordinate in status to doctors and Pollard (2011, p. 613) has suggested that the rise in 'medicine during the nineteenth century as a rational "masculine science" has resulted in the irrational "feminine" being pathologised'. The increasing dominance of obstetric-led care and technological intervention ensured that birth was perceived to be a risky business that needed to be closely controlled and managed in order to protect both the mother and baby from harm. Such views encouraged the destabilisation of the role of midwives in promoting normal birth and validated hospitals as being the safest places to give birth.

While it is important to be aware of the significant advantages that such advances in technology may bring through its judicious use upon an informed and appropriately selected population, it is the widespread indiscriminate use of such technology and the medical 'management' of birth that has served to increase intervention during birth along with its associated morbidity and mortality. There has been much published literature relating to the control of childbirth by technology and medicalisation and Hunter and Segrott (2014) have suggested how the history of midwifery can provide insight into the historical underpinnings of the tensions that exist between some midwives and doctors today as they struggle for **occupational jurisdiction**.

Trigger

Debates about **medicalised** and **naturalised childbirth** are often polarised between these two distinct factions, when often the reality exists somewhere in between.

Think about five examples where technology has been beneficial for childbearing women and their families and helped to save life and prevent morbidity and mortality.

Table 2.1 Summary of the key findings of the national
survey of women's experience of maternity care as
compared with earlier findings

Areas that need to improve still	Areas that had improved
Information and support are being provided inconsistently. Information needed to make choices was not consistently provided and the choices themselves were not universally offered to women. Fewer women reported that they were not left alone during labour or birth at a time that worried them. Almost one in five women felt that their concerns during labour were not taken seriously.	The proportion of women who said that they were always spoken to in a way they could understand during antenatal care and labour and birth was increased from the previous survey. More women felt that they were always involved during antenatal care and labour and birth. More women felt that they were treated with kindness and understanding and had confidence and trust in the staff caring for them during labour and birth.

Source: Adapted from CQC, 2013

Whereas the rhetoric about the importance of continuity of care, choice and control for all women during their childbearing experience persists, the reality of midwifery practice today often remains somewhat different. The Commission for Healthcare Audit and Inspection (The Healthcare Commission) was replaced in 2009 by the Care Quality Commission (CQC) as the independent regulator of health and social care in England. The CQC regulates the provision of health and adult care services across England to check that standards are being met. The results of their latest survey (CQC, 2013), which looked at the experiences of people receiving maternity services in England, found that although there was evidence of improvements since their last survey (CQC, 2010) there were still several areas where there was no improvement and women's experiences continued to fall short of their expectations. These are summarised within Table 2.1.

The CQC has also been instrumental in identifying serious failings within the maternity care provided at several hospitals following the public inquiry into the Mid-Staffordshire NHS Foundation Trust led by Robert Francis. The Francis report (Francis, 2013) was produced in response to the severe concerns and failings highlighted regarding the quality and safety of the care provided to those using the service. Its recommendations included the urgent need for organisations to create and maintain the right culture to deliver high-quality care that is responsive to patients' needs and preferences, thus making explicit the link between **organisational culture** and the safety and performance of an organisation (see Box 2.3).

Leadership is crucial to improving both the organisation and culture within hospitals and maternity units and several key documents have highlighted this (Ham, 2014). While from a macro perspective there is a need for organisations to be built on sound

---

Box 2.3   Overview of the negative aspects of the culture identified in the Francis report

- A lack of openness to criticism and defensiveness
- A lack of consideration to patients
- Misplaced assumptions about the judgements and actions of others
- An acceptance of poor standards
- A failure to put the patient first in everything that is done

Source: Francis, 2013

---

structures with a clear corporate and strategic leadership (Department of Health, 2000), it is paramount that urgent attention is also paid to the micro perspective. The various interprofessional relationships that exist and contribute to the culture within maternity units have an enormous influence upon the care that is provided to childbearing women (Frith et al, 2014) and individual practitioner behaviour (Hastie and Fahy, 2011). The provision of substandard communication between professionals has also been identified as a significant contributory factor to maternal deaths (Centre for Maternal and Child Enquiries, 2011; Knight et al., 2014).

Whereas it is evident from a historical perspective that there are fundamental clinical and professional differences between midwives and physicians with regards to maternity care, recent findings suggest that these differences may also 'become viral, resulting in a general (and self-perpetuating) expectation among midwives and medical staff that collaboration is likely to be difficult' (Downe et al., 2010, p. 251). Davis-Floyd (2003) has suggested that there are two basic opposing models of birth available to pregnant women within our society and these are the technocratic model of birth associated mainly with medicine that considers birth as an inherently dangerous process, and the holistic model of birth associated mainly with midwifery and where birth is considered as a social event based on normal physiological processes. However it is too simplistic to categorise practitioners as subscribing to either of these two approaches and Pollard (2011) suggests instead that maternity care be hypothesised as a continuum with one of these approaches at either end and along which practitioners inhabit a range of positions.

More recently midwifery is seeking to increase its professional terrain and renegotiate its boundaries and relationships with doctors (Hunter and Segrott, 2014). Midwifery-focused skills that have historically been undervalued within practice in favour of scientific technology have become reaffirmed and recognised as important in ensuring women are **empowered** to optimise their birthing experience (RCM, 2007). Such skills include the provision of emotional support, encouraging women to mobilise and adopt different positions during labour and participate in non-pharmacological pain relieving strategies where appropriate. Research has highlighted the benefits that **midwifery-led care** provides to childbearing women (Cragin and Kennedy, 2006;

Hatem et al., 2008) and maternity units are required to put systems and guidelines in place to ensure that midwifery-led care is provided for those women with uncomplicated pregnancies and birth. The publication of clear guidance is important in order to reduce the morbidity associated with unnecessary intervention while also ensuring that those women with identified medical and/or obstetric risk factors are referred appropriately for obstetric-led care.

Government documents highlight the importance of ensuring visible clinical midwifery leadership both in practice and in the development of policies and strategies to develop and improve maternity care (Department of Health, 1999, 2009; NHS Executive, 1998). The role of the **consultant midwife** is now well established within England and an established consultant midwife training programme has been provided in some part of the UK since 2008. This is to ensure that opportunity is provided for midwives to acquire the appropriate skills and professional development in areas such as strategic leadership, service improvement and policy.

The recommendations of the Francis report and the literature that has since been generated emphasises the importance of all staff having clear objectives, shared values, openness to improvement initiatives and to feel appreciated and respected (West et al., 2011). This can be achieved partly through engaging midwives, doctors and other staff in improvement programmes (Ham, 2014) and multidisciplinary training. The provision of care needs to be evidence based and support the wishes of women and their families while ensuring that sufficient information has been provided to facilitate decision making with regards to care choices. Such principles are reflected in the NMC Code (NMC, 2015), which sets out the principles to which midwives and nurses should adhere.

Despite this and as history has shown, a dichotomy may occur where national and professional guidance, stipulating the need to promote a positive working culture and enhance opportunities for normal birth, is failing to be translated into practice at grass-roots level. As we have already noted, this can be seen through examples of where long-standing medicalised practice *continues* to be routinely implemented within delivery suites, *despite* the evidence that now exists that reveals that such practices are not beneficial to all women and may even increase the likelihood of unnecessary intervention. In Box 2.4 there is an overview of some examples of these routine practices.

Box 2.4   An overview of some examples of medical/midwifery practices that continue to persist in some units despite evidence that shows they are not beneficial and may be harmful to women and their babies

Directive pushing during the second stage of labour for women who do not have an epidural (Byrom and Downe, 2005; Cooke, 2010; Prins et al., 2011; Walsh, 2007)

(continued)

(continued)

Admission CTG or CTGs for women who do not have a clinical indication that predisposes the fetus to hypoxia (for e.g. previous fourth degree tear, previous postpartum haemorrhage) (Alfirevic et al., 2013)

Immobility during labour (de Jonge et al., 2004; Gupta et al, 2012)

Women without a medical or obstetric risk factor labouring and giving birth on the delivery suite (Birthplace in England Collaborative Group, 2011)

Lack of effective support during labour or failure to facilitate support from the woman's birth partner (Hodnett et al., 2007)

Dilemmas can arise for midwives in practice when endeavouring to negotiate the culture within which they work, follow local guidelines and professional regulations. Often there are areas of conflict where midwives are required to offer women information to enable informed decisions to be made and to support women in their birth choices (NMC, 2015). This may on occasions directly conflict with both the culture and busyness of a unit where minimal time is available for discussion with women and hospital policies and guidelines may not always facilitate woman-centred care.

Application to practice

Consider the example of a woman who previously suffered a traumatic birth resulting in an emergency caesarean section. In hindsight she feels that this may partly be due to the fact that she was unable to move around during labour and consented to epidural analgesia. For this pregnancy she is keen to do things differently and would like to use the pool on the delivery suite and be as mobile as possible.

What are the dilemmas that a midwife may face when supporting a woman with her choice? How might the midwife **advocate** for women while ensuring that evidence-based care is provided? What support strategies are available to midwives to help them with this?

Often the practices outlined within Box 2.4 are enforced by midwives, and Kirkham (1999) has suggested that oppressed groups often internalise the values of those in power and reject their own principles and identity. In this way midwives working within a medicalised environment may internalise the values of the medicalised model of birth (Hunter, 2004, 2005) and subscribe to a more interventionist model of care so that interventions within childbirth become accepted practice at the expense of midwifery **autonomy** and the provision of **woman-centred care**.

Trigger

There is a lot of literature that discusses the **iatrogenic** complications of childbirth or the cascade of intervention whereby intervention during labour or childbirth results in further intervention along with its associated increased morbidity for women.

Box 2.4 provides some examples of medical/midwifery practices that continue to persist, despite evidence that shows they are not beneficial and may be harmful to women and their babies. Can you think of any other examples from practice? What strategies might be taken to promote and optimise opportunities for normal birth within your unit?

Recent evidence also shows that midwives may practice covertly in order to support women's choices and promote normal birth (Bluff and Holloway, 2008) or seek to obey and conform to the predominant model of care and cultural norm within which they work. Current approaches to managing risk, while vital in ensuring safe care when used appropriately and judiciously, also have the potential to **disempower** both midwives and the women in their care when used inappropriately to promote and sustain a culture of fear around childbirth.

Although it is beyond the constraints of this chapter to explore the nature of risk in full, midwives should be aware of the language that they employ to ensure that they are not inadvertently using it to steer women (Levy, 2006) in the direction that the midwife rather than the woman chooses. Such strategies may be undertaken by midwives who are anxious about challenging established practices and lack the time for a full discussion with women to promote informed choice. As always it is important to get the balance right. Ensuring a safe culture involves having respectful dialogues with colleagues to ensure that the care provided is evidence based and to minimise risks of associated morbidity and mortality from unnecessary intervention, as well as ensuring that women with established medical and obstetric risk factors are offered appropriate referral, assessment and obstetric-led care.

Trigger

How might you try to 'control' a situation within midwifery practice because of time constraints or concerns? Think about the booking interview, presenting options around place of birth and the way that you might present information. What are the factors that influence the information that you choose to give to women?

The Kings Fund (2014) undertook a survey to review the culture within the NHS and found that only 39 per cent of staff surveyed (n=2030) felt that their organisation was characterised by openness, transparency and challenge. Various initiatives have since been implemented both at local and national levels and the Kings Fund's *Improving Services in Maternity Services* (a toolkit for teams) (Thomas and Dixon, 2012) has identified a number of approaches designed to help increase the safety of maternity services. These include the development of effective communication strategies and teamwork among staff and initiatives undertaken to challenge interprofessional and departmental barriers.

The supervision of midwives and consultant midwives' role has the potential to challenge poor organisational culture, advocate for childbearing women and their families, support midwives and promote high standards of practice and woman-centred care (see Box 2.5). However such roles are often only as effective as the organisational structure within which they operate and can potentially serve to perpetuate the very culture they are intended to change. Varying discourses of childbirth may serve to reinforce segregated values and ways of working but there is a need for a joined-up approach within maternity care among professionals that values both midwifery-led skills and obstetric expertise within complicated childbirth and birth.

Box 2.5   Overview of midwifery supervision

The Nursing and Midwifery Order (Stationery Office, 2001) requires the establishment of a local supervising authority (LSA) for midwifery in every geographical area and requires midwives to give notice of their intention to practise in that area (Parliamentary and Health Service Ombudsman, 2013). Each LSA must ensure the supervision of all midwives in their area and investigate any concerns about midwives' practice. The stated purpose of the supervision of midwives is to protect women and babies by actively promoting a safe standard of midwifery practice (NMC, 2009). For midwifery, supervision is a statutory responsibility that also aims to provide a mechanism for support and guidance. Strengths of supervision include the support for midwives and women that it provides through 24-hour access to an on-call supervisor of midwives.

The childbearing woman and her family

Women's experiences of childbirth are profoundly related to the lives of women in society and there have been several changes within society that have impacted upon the population of childbearing women.

Over the past decade there has been an increasing trend towards women having babies later in life and between 2001 and 2012 the number of babies born in England to women aged 40 or over rose by 85 per cent (up 13,280) (RCM, 2013). The reasons motherhood is postponed are various and multifaceted. Common reasons may include: to achieve financial independence, to build a career, to pursue further education and be in an established relationship with a supportive partner. Adverse pregnancy outcomes

---

Box 2.6 Overview of trends in the maternal population in England

- The total fertility rate has fallen with an average of 1.85 children per woman in 2013 (largest annual decrease since 1975)
- Increase in births outside of marriage and civil partnership
- Increase in births to mothers born outside of the UK
- Increase in women over 40 giving birth
- Decrease in teenagers giving birth
- Increase in the complexity of births

Source: Adapted from RCM, 2013 and ONS, 2013

---

also rise with age, and women over 40 are considered to be at a higher risk of pregnancy complications (Delpisheh et al., 2008; Joseph et al., 2005; Royal Collage of Obstetricians and Gynaecologists, 2009). However it is important to remember that most pregnancies will result in a healthy baby (Royal Collage of Obstetricians and Gynaecologists, 2009) and women should be supported in their choices about their childbearing.

Such changes are reflective of broader sociological perspectives and can be viewed within the context of a United Kingdom society characterised by falling fertility rates and increased levels of childlessness, as recent years have shown that less women are having children. In 2012, around one in five women (born in 1967) in England and Wales had never had children, compared with their mother's generation (born in 1940) where one in nine had never had children (ONS, 2013). The last 15 years has also seen a change in the living arrangements of young adults, with 26 per cent of adults in the UK aged between 20 and 34 years living with a parent or parents in 2013 (ONS, 2013.) This shows an increase of 25 per cent since 1996, despite the number of people in the population aged 20 to 34 being largely the same in 1996 and 2013 (ONS, 2013). Such findings may reflect how factors such as increasing participation in higher education, increased house prices and living costs and job insecurity may result in adults remaining at their parents' home for longer out of financial necessity (Stone et al., 2011; Wilcox, 2008).

A trend towards having smaller families is also apparent and the total fertility rate has fallen with an average of 1.85 children per woman in 2013 (ONS, 2013). Browne (2011) has suggested that such changes demonstrate the reduced function of the family, where roles such as childcare that were originally undertaken by the mother are transferred to other social institutions such as nurseries and child minders.

The current government has tried to reinforce the role of the family by stating that strong families are the bedrock of society (Conservative Party, 2010). There has also been an increased focus on the role of children within society and government initiatives to improve the quality of lives for children have resulted in legislation that ensures that child care has come under increasing scrutiny (Children's Rights Alliance for England, 2013; Department for Children, Schools and Families/Department of Health, 2009). As a result of this, children's lives have become progressively contained and in many ways constrained as planned educational and recreational activities are provided for them (Browne, 2011).

The role of the media and emergence of new technology in the late-twentieth and early-twenty-first centuries has played a significant part in defining women's expectations about pregnancy and childbirth (Hall, 2013). Romano et al. (2010) have stated that social media has the ability to shift the power between producers and consumers by enabling the sharing of interactive information. Media has become interactive and is no longer one dimensional as childbearing women and their partners are able to engage in online discussions, share experiences and provide support and advice.

Trigger

Consider how you use mass media. What information are women able to access? How accurate do you think this information is?

Lagan et al. (2010) sought to ascertain why and how pregnant women use the Internet as a health information source, and the overall effect it had on their decision making and found that the Internet played a significant part in the respondents' health information seeking and decision making in pregnancy. In a further study Lagan et al. (2011) aimed to explore women's experiences and perceptions of using the Internet for retrieving pregnancy-related information, and its influence on their decision-making processes. Again the Internet appeared to have a visible impact on women's decision making in relation to all aspects of pregnancy and women found that they were able to validate information, share experience and feel empowered with the choices that they made. Thus the Internet and social media have become a valuable source of information for women and Lagan et al. (2011) have emphasised the need for health professionals to work in partnership with women to guide them toward evidence-based websites and to be prepared to discuss the ensuing information.

Couldry (2012) has described today's media and information revolution as being comparable in depth to and even faster than the print revolution and highlights how this has resulted in an exponential growth of data volume, where whole sectors of public and professional life are being transformed by the changes in information production. However Ofcom (2011) has found that although take-up among all groups has recently increased, younger people, men and those in higher socioeconomic groups are more likely to have access to the Internet at home. It is important that the increase in use of online technology to provide information does not supersede more traditional methods of information giving such as leaflets and face-to-face discussion. This is to ensure that those women who are socially disadvantaged and without immediate means to online connection do not become further excluded from maternity care. Couldry (2012) has also cautioned against the forms of disconnection that may emerge with increased media usage, whereby the online world is assumed to be a universal reference point, thus excluding those without the immediate means to online connection.

It is clear that within today's society there remains a significantly large vulnerable and differentiated population of childbearing women and families. The impact of domestic violence is widespread with the *Local Crime Survey* revealing that within England and Wales 7 per cent of women and 4 per cent of men were estimated to have experienced domestic abuse in 2012/2013 (ONS, 2014). This is equivalent to around 1.2 million female and 700,000 male victims. The survey also found that 1 in 10 respondents felt that it was mostly or sometimes acceptable to hit or slap their partner in response to their partner having an affair, thus demonstrating that aggression and violence to women is part of the accepted behaviour in some relationships.

Pregnancy is a particularly vulnerable time for women as abuse is likely to start or escalate during pregnancy (Home Office, 2009; Steen and Keeling, 2012). The term 'domestic abuse' has been redefined and also covers issues that may concern women from minority ethnic backgrounds, such as female genital mutilation and forced marriage (Department of Health, 2006b). Previous confidential enquiry reports into maternal deaths have highlighted the issue of domestic abuse and drawn attention to the features of poor attendance and late booking to maternity care associated with those mothers who died (Lewis, 2007). These associations have decreased more recently (Centre for Maternal and Child Enquiries, 2011; Knight et al., 2014) and may demonstrate the effectiveness of some of the government-driven recommendations that have since been put in place. However it is important that healthcare professionals do not become complacent and the Centre for Maternal and Child Enquiries (2011) continued to recommend that midwives should ensure that all women are seen alone at least once during the antenatal period to facilitate disclosure of domestic abuse and high priority should be given to routine enquiry about whether women are suffering from abuse.

Within England and Wales the infant mortality rate continues to fall. In 2011, there were 4.2 infant deaths per 1,000 live births, which is the lowest rate on record (ONS, 2013). This is a 62 per cent decrease from the 11.1 infant deaths per 1,000 live births in 1981 (ONS, 2013). However despite this it is evident that social disparities and inequalities that exist before birth can impact on pregnancy, including maternal and perinatal death and can persist across generations (Acheson, 1998; Spencer, 2008). Infant mortality rates are worse in disadvantaged groups and areas and poor health outcomes are often linked to social factors such as education, work, income and the environment (Department of Health, 2010). Ethnicity and deprivation continue to be significantly associated with adverse maternal and perinatal outcomes, which include stillbirth and neonatal death and the last confidential enquiry found that women with partners who were unemployed or whose jobs were unclassified were nearly six times more likely to die from maternal causes than women with husbands or partners in employment (Centre for Maternal and Child Enquiries, 2011). Overall findings have shown that although a significant disparity remains, the measures of inequality appear to be reducing in response to government-driven initiatives that maternity services have put in place to provide care for vulnerable women.

Conclusion

This chapter has introduced the reader to an overview of the history and regulation of midwifery and the social and organisational factors that impact upon maternity services. It has critically evaluated the midwife's role today and encouraged the reader to consider how a positive working culture can be established to facilitate the promotion of professional relations and women-centred care. A brief overview of the recent changes within society and their potential impact upon the population of childbearing women has also been presented.

Overall recent advances in technology have improved information access for most women and theoretically enabled greater choice with regards to decisions to be made concerning childrearing and childbirth. While ensuring that midwives continue to maintain and promote their skills in optimising opportunity for normal birth, there is also a need to recognise the value of appropriately used technological skill in the face of the changing population of women giving birth. Thus a collaborative approach is required for maternity care whereby the skills of all birth professionals are valued and clear processes and structures are in place that facilitate women's choice and ensure that women are able to make choices about the most appropriate options for their care.

References

Acheson, D. (1998) *Inequalities in Health: Report of an independent inquiry.* London: HMSO

AIMS (Association for Improvements in the Maternity Services) (2010) *What is Aims?* Online at: http://www.aims.org.uk/whatisaims.htm Accessed 1 July 2014

Alfirevic, Z., Devane, D. and Gyte, G.M.L. (2013) Continuous cardiotocography (CTG) as a form of electronic fetal monitoring (EFM) for fetal assessment during labour. *Cochrane Database of Systematic Reviews* 2013, Issue 5. Art. No.: CD006066. DOI:10.1002/14651858.CD006066.pub2.

Benoit, C., Wrede, S., Bourgeault, I., Sandall, J., De Vries, R. and van Teijlingen, E. R. (2005) Understanding the social organisation of maternity care systems: midwifery as a touchstone. *Sociology of Health & Illness* Volume 27, No. 6, pp. 722–737.

Berg, M. and Dahlberg, K. (1998) A phenomenological study of women's experiences of complicated childbirth. *Midwifery* Volume 14, pp. 23–29

Berg, M., Lundgren, I., Hermansson, E. and Wahlberg, V. (1996) Women's experience of the encounter with the midwife during childbirth. *Midwifery* Volume 12, pp. 11–15

Birthplace in England Collaborative Group (2011) Perinatal and maternal outcomes by planned place of birth for healthy women with low risk pregnancies: the Birthplace in England national prospective cohort study. *BMJ* 343:d7400. Online at: http://www.bmj.com/content/343/bmj.d7400 Accessed 4 July 2014

Bluff, R. and Holloway, I. (2008) The efficacy of midwifery role models. *Midwifery* Volume 24, pp. 301–09

Borrelli, S. E. (2013) What is a good midwife? Some historical considerations. *Evidence Based Midwifery* Volume 11, No. 2, pp. 51–59

Browne, K. (2011) *An Introduction to Sociology.* Fourth Edition. Cambridge: Polity Press

Byrom, A. and Downe, S. (2005) Second stage of labour: Challenging the use of directed pushing. *RCM Midwives* Volume 8, No. 4, pp. 168–69

Centre for Maternal and Child Enquiries (2011) Saving Mothers' Lives Reviewing maternal deaths to make motherhood safer: 2006–2008. The Eighth Report of the Confidential Enquiries into Maternal Deaths in the United Kingdom. *BJOG* Volume 118 (Supplement 1) pp. 1–203

Chalmers, I., Enkin, M. and Keirse, M. J. (1989) *Effective Care in Pregnancy and Childbirth.* Oxford: Oxford University Press

Children's Rights Alliance for England (2013) *State of Children's Rights in England: Government action on United Nations' recommendations for strengthening children's rights in the UK.* London: CRAE. Online: http://www.crae.org.uk/media/64143/CRAE_England_Report_WEB.pdf Accessed 6 July 2014

Conservative Party (2010) *Invitation to Join the Government of Britain.* Online: http://www.conservatives.com/~/media/files/activist%20centre/press%20and%20policy/manifestos/manifesto2010 Accessed 20 July 2014

Cooke, A. (2010) When will we change practice and stop directive pushing in labour? *British Journal of Midwifery* Volume 8, No. 2, pp. 78–81

Couldry, N. (2012) *Media, Society, World: Social theory and digital media practice.* Cambridge: Polity Press

CQC (Care Quality Commission) (2010) *Women's Experiences of Maternity Care in England: Key findings from the 2010 NHS trust survey.* Online: http://www.cqc.org.uk/sites/default/files/documents/20101201_mat10_briefing_final_for_publication_201101072550.pdf Accessed 4 July 2014

CQC (2013) *National Findings from the 2013 Survey of Women's Experiences of Maternity Care.* Online: http://www.cqc.org.uk/sites/default/files/documents/maternity_report_for_publication.pdf Accessed 4 July 2014

Cragin, L. and Kennedy, H. P. (2006) Linking obstetric and midwifery practice with optimal outcomes. *Journal of Obstetric, Gynaecologic, & Neonatal Nursing* Volume 5, No. 6, pp. 779–85

Davis-Floyd, R. E. (2003) *Birth as an American Rite of Passage.* Second Edition. Berkeley: University of California Press

Davis-Floyd, R. E. and Sargeant, C. F (1997) *Childbirth and Authorative Knowledge – Cross cultural perspectives.* California: University of California Press

Davis, A. (2013) *Choice, Policy and Practice in Maternity Care since 1948.* Online: http://www.historyandpolicy.org/policy-papers/papers/choice-policy-and-practice-in-maternity-care-since-1948 Accessed 4 July 2014

De Jonge, A., Teunissen, T. A. M. and Lagro-Janssen, A. L. M. (2004) Supine position compared to other positions during the second stage of labor: A meta-analytic review. *Journal of Psychosomatic Obstetrics & Gynecology* Volume 25, No. 1, pp. 35–45

Delpisheh, A., Brabin, L., Attia, E. and Brabin, B. J. (2008) Pregnancy late in life: a hospital-based study of birth outcomes. *Journal of Women's Health* Volume 17, No. 6, pp. 965–70

Department for Children, Schools and Families/ Department of Health (2009) *Healthy Lives, Brighter Futures: The strategy for children and young people's health.* London: Crown Copyright

Department of Health (1993) *Changing Childbirth: Report of the Expert Maternity Group.* London: Crown Copyright

Department of Health (1999) *Saving Lives: Our Healthier Nation.* London: Stationery Office

Department of Health (2000) *An Organisation with a Memory.* London: Crown Copy Right. Online: http://www.aagbi.org/sites/default/files/An%20organisation%20with%20a%20memory.pdf Accessed 1 April 2014

Department of Health (2006a) *National Guidelines for Maternity Services Liaison Committees (MSLCs)*. London: Crown Copyright

Department of Health (2006b) *Responding to Domestic Abuse. A Handbook for Health Professionals*. London: Department of Health

Department of Health (2007) *Maternity Matters: Choice, Access and Continuity of Care in a Safe Service*. London: Crown Copyright

Department of Health (2009) *Delivering High Quality Midwifery Care: The priorities opportunities and challenges for midwives*. London: Crown Copyright

Department of Health (2010) *Tackling Health Inequalities in Infant and Maternal Health Outcomes – Report of the Infant Mortality National Support Team*. London: Department of Health

DHSS (Department of Health and Social Security) (1972) *Report of the Committee on Nursing*. London: HMSO

Dodwell, M. and Newburn, M. (2010) *Normal Birth as a Measure of the Quality of Care: Evidence on safety, effectiveness and women's experiences*. London: National Childbirth Trust

Donnison, J. (1988) *Midwives and Medical Men: A history of the struggle for the control of childbirth*. London: Historical publications

Downe, S., Finlayson, K. and Fleming, A. (2010) Creating a collaborative culture in maternity care. *Journal of Midwifery and Women's Health* Volume 55, No. 3, pp. 250–54

Francis, R. (2013) *Report of the Mid-Staffordshire NHS Foundation Trust Public Inquiry*. London: HMSO

Frith, L., Sinclair, M., Vehviläinen-Julkunen, K., Beeckman, K., Loytved, C. and Luyben, A. (2014) Organisational culture in maternity care: A scoping review. *Evidence Based Midwifery* Volume 12, No. 1, pp. 16–22

Graham, I. D. (1997) *Episiotomy: Challenging Obstetric Interventions*. Oxford: Blackwell Science

Graham, I. D., Logan, J., Davies, B. and Nimrod, C. (2004) Changing the use of electronic fetal monitoring and labor support: A case study of barriers and facilitators. *Birth* Volume 31, No. 4, pp. 293–301

Green, J. M. and Baston, H. (2003) Feeling in control during labour: concepts, correlates and consequences. *Birth* Volume 30, No. 4, pp. 235–47

Green, J. M., Baston, H., Easton, S. and McCormick, F. (2003) *Greater Expectations? Inter-relationships between women's expectations and experiences of decision making, continuity, choice and control in labour, and psychological outcomes: a summary report*. Leeds: Mother and Infant Research Unit. Online: http://www.york.ac.uk/media/healthsciences/documents/miru/GreaterExpdf.pdf Accessed 20 July 2014

Gupta, J. K., Hofmeyr, G. J. and Shehmar, M. (2012) Position in the second stage of labour for women without epidural anaesthesia. *Cochrane Database of Systematic Reviews* 2012, Issue 5. Art. No.: CD002006. DOI: 10.1002/14651858.CD002006.pub

Hall, J. G. (2013) As seen on TV: Media influences on pregnancy and pre-birth narratives. In Ryan, K. M. and Macey, D. A. (eds) *Television and the Self: Knowledge Identity and Media Representation*. Plymouth: Lexington Books, pp. 47–62

Hall, S. and Holloway, I. (1998) Staying in control. Women's experiences of labour in water. *Midwifery* Volume 14 No. 1, pp. 30–36

Ham, C. (2014) *Reforming the NHS From Within: Beyond hierarchy, inspection and markets*. London: The Kings Fund. Online: http://www.kingsfund.org.uk/sites/files/kf/field/field_publication_file/reforming-the-nhs-from-within-kingsfund-jun14.pdf Accessed 4 July 2014

Hastie, C. and Fahy, K. (2011) Inter-professional collaboration in delivery suite: A qualitative study. *Women & Birth: Journal of the Australian College of Midwives* Volume 24 No. 2, pp. 72– 79

Hatem, M., Sandall, J., Devane, D., Soltani, H. and Gates, S. (2008) Midwife-led versus other models of care for childbearing women. *Cochrane Database of Systematic Reviews* 4: CD004667. DOI: 10.1002/14651858.CD004667.pub2

Hodnett, E. D., Gates, S., Hofmeyr, G. J. and Sakala, C. (2007) Continuous support for women during childbirth. *Cochrane Database of Systematic Reviews* 2012, Issue 10. Art. No.: CD003766. DOI: 10.1002/14651858.CD003766.pub4

Home Office (2009) *British Crime Survey 2008–09*. London: HMSO

Hunter, B. (2004) Conflicting ideologies as a source of emotion work in midwifery. *Midwifery* Volume 20, pp. 261–72

Hunter, B. (2005) Emotion work and boundary maintenance in hospital based midwifery. *Midwifery* Volume 21, pp. 253–66

Hunter, B. and Segrott, J. (2014) Renegotiating inter-professional boundaries in maternity care: Implementing a clinical pathway for normal labour. *Sociology of Health and Illness* Volume 36, No. 5, pp. 719–37

Joseph, K. S., Allen, A. C., Dodds, L., Turner, L. A., Scott, H. and Liston, R. (2005) The perinatal effects of delayed childbearing. *Obstetrics & Gynaecology* Volume 105, No. 6, pp. 1410–18

Kings Fund (2014) *Culture and Leadership in the NHS – The Kings Fund Survey*. London: Kings Fund. Online: http://www.kingsfund.org.uk/sites/files/kf/field/field_publication_file/survey-culture-leadership-nhs-may2014.pdf Accessed 20 July 2014

Kirkham, M. (1999) The culture of midwifery in the NHS in England. *Journal of Advanced Nursing* Volume 30, No. 3, pp. 732–39

Knight, M., Kenyon, S., Brocklehurst, P., Neilson, J., Shakespeare, J. and Kurinczuk, J. J. (eds) (2014) on behalf of MBRRACE-UK. *Saving Lives, Improving Mothers' Care: Lessons learned to inform future maternity care from the UK and Ireland Confidential Enquiries into Maternal Deaths and Morbidity 2009–2012*. Oxford: National Perinatal Epidemiology Unit, University of Oxford

Lagan, B. M., Sinclair, M. and Kernohan, W. G. (2010) Internet use in pregnancy informs women's decision making: A web-based survey. *Birth* Volume 37, No. 2, pp. 106–15

Lagan, B. M., Sinclair, M. and Kernohan, W. G. (2011) What is the impact of the Internet on decision-making in pregnancy? A global study. *Birth* Volume 38, No. 4, pp. 336–45

Leap, N. and Hunter, B. (1993) *The Midwife's Tale. An oral history from handywoman to professional midwife*. London: Scarlett Press

Levy, V. (2006) Protective steering: A grounded theory study of the processes by which midwives facilitate informed choices during pregnancy. *Journal of Advanced Nursing* Volume 53, No. 1, pp. 114–22

Lewis, G. (2007). *Saving Mother's Lives: Reviewing Maternal Deaths to Make Motherhood Safer. 2003–05. The Seventh Report of the Confidential Enquiries into Maternal Deaths in the United Kingdom*. London: RCOG

Mayes, M. (1930) *An Introduction to Midwifery. Elementary anatomy, physiology and antenatal hygiene*. London: Faber and Faber

NHS (National Health Service) Executive (1998) A Consultation on a Strategy for Nursing, Midwifery and Health Visiting. *Health Service Circular (HSC) 1998/045*. London: HMSO

Nightingale, F. (1871) *Introductory notes on lying-in institutions together with a proposal for organizing an institution for training midwives and midwifery nurses*. London: Longmans Green and Company

NMC (Nursing Midwifery Council) (2009) *Modern Supervision in Action*. London: NMC

NMC (2010) *The history of Nursing and Midwifery Regulation*. (Updated 2014). Online: http://www.nmc-uk.org/about-us/the-history-of-nursing-and-midwifery-regulation/ Accessed 23 July 2014

NMC (2012) *Midwives Rules and Standards.* London: NMC

NMC (2015) *The Code. Professional Standards of Practice and Behaviour for Nurses and Midwives.* London: NMC. Online: http://www.nmc-uk.org/Documents/NMC-Publications/NMC-Code-A5-FINAL.pdf last accessed February 2015

Nuttall, A. (2012) Midwifery, 1800–1920: The journey to registration. In Borsay, A. and Hunter, B. (eds) *Nursing and Midwifery in Britain.* Basingstoke: Palgrave Macmillan, pp. 128–150

Ofcom (Independent regulator and competition authority for the UK communications industries) (2011) *Home Internet Access: By age, socio-economic group and gender.* Online: http://stakeholders.ofcom.org.uk/market-data-research/market-data/communications-market-reports/cmr11/internet-web/4.17 Accessed 20 July 2014

ONS (Office for National Statistics) (2012) *Births in England and Wales by Characteristics of Birth 2, 2012. Online*: http://www.ons.gov.uk/ons/rel/vsob1/characteristics-of-birth-2—england-and-wales/2012/sb-characteristics-of-birth-2.html Accessed 20 July 2014

ONS (2013) *Characteristic of Mothers, England and Wales.* Online: http://www.ons.gov.uk/ons/rel/vsob1/characteristics-of-Mother-1—england-and-wales/index.html Accessed 20 July 2014

ONS (2014*) Crime Statistics, Focus on Violent Crime and Sexual Offences, 2012/13.* Online: http://www.ons.gov.uk/ons/rel/crime-stats/crime-statistics/index.html Accessed 20 July 2014

Parliament (1902) *The Midwives Act 1902.* London: HMSO

Parliament (1979) *Nurses, Midwives and Health Visitors Act 1979.* Online: http://www.legislation.gov.uk/ukpga/1979/36/pdfs/ukpga_19790036_en.pdf Accessed 20 July 2014

Parliamentary and Health Service Ombudsman (2013) *Midwifery Supervision and Regulation: Recommendations for change.* London: The Stationery Office

Pollard, K. C. (2011) How midwives' discursive practices contribute to the maintenance of the status quo in English maternity care. *Midwifery* Volume 27, pp. 612–19

Prins, M., Boxem, J., Lucas, C. and Hutton, E.(2011) Effect of spontaneous pushing versus Valsalva pushing in the second stage of labour on mother and fetus: a systematic review of randomised trials. *BJOG* Volume 118, pp. 662–70

Romano, A. M., Gerber, H. and Andrews, D. (2010) Social media, power and the future of VBAC. *The Journal of Perinatal Education* Volume 19 No. 3, pp. 43–52

RCM (Royal College of Midwives) (n.d.) *Archive Hub – Records of the Royal College of Midwives.* Online: http://archiveshub.ac.uk/data/gb1538-rcm Accessed 25 July 2014

RCM (2007) *Normal Childbirth – position statement no. 4.* Online: https://www.rcm.org.uk/sites/default/files/POSITION%20STATEMENT%20Normal-Childbirth.pdf Accessed 20 July 2014

RCM (2013) *State of the Maternity Services Report 2013.* London: RCM

Royal College of Obstetricians and Gynaecologists (2009) *RCOG Statement on Later Maternal Age.* Online: http://www.rcog.org.uk/what-we-do/campaigning-and-opinions/statement/rcog-statement-later-maternal-age Accessed 20 July 2014

Royal College of Obstetricians and Gynaecologists (2012) *From the Archive: International Women's Day 2012.* Online: http://www.rcog.org.uk/what-we-do/information-services/-collections/-archive-international-womens-day-2012 Accessed 20 July 2014

Royal College of Obstetricians and Gynaecologists Heritage Collections Blog (2013) *Midwives Chronicle and Nursing Notes, November 1979.* Online: http://rcmheritage.wordpress.com/tag/midwives-and-health-visitors-act/ Accessed 20 July 2014

Sakala, C. and Corry, M. P. (2008) *Evidence-Based Maternity Care: What It Is and What It Can Achieve.* Childbirth Connection, the Reforming States Group, and the Milbank

Memorial Fund. Online: http://www.milbank.org/uploads/documents/0809Maternity Care/0809MaternityCare.html Accessed 4 July 2014

Spencer, N. (2008) *Health Consequences of Poverty for Children. End Child Poverty.* Online: http://www.endchildpoverty.org.uk/news/publications/child-poverty-an d-health—supplementary-chapter-2/26/123 Accessed 14 November 2014

Standing Maternity and Midwifery Advisory Committee (1970) *Domiciliary Midwifery and Maternity Bed Needs.* Report of the sub-committee. Chairman: Sir John Peel. London: HMSO

Stationery Office (2002) *The Nursing and Midwifery Order 2001.* Statutory Instrument 2002 No 253. London: HMSO. Online: www.opsi.gov.uk/si/si2002/20020253.htm Accessed 20 July 2014

Steen, M. and Keeling, J. (2012) Stop! Silent screams. *The Practising Midwife* 15 No. 2, pp. 28–30

Stone, J., Berrington, A. and Falkingham J. (2011) The changing determinants of UK young adults' living arrangements. *Demographic Research* Volume 25, Article 20, pp. 629–66. Online: http://www.demographic-research.org/Volumes/Vol25/20/ DOI: 10.4054/ DemRes.2011.25.20 Accessed 20 November 2014

Symonds, A. and Hunt, S. (1996) *The Midwife and Society: Perspectives, policies and practice.* Hampshire: Macmillan Press

Tew, M. (1985) Place of birth and perinatal mortality. *Journal of the Royal College of General Practitioners* Volume 35, pp. 390–94

Tew, M. (1998) *Safer Childbirth? A critical history of maternity care.* London: Free Association Books Ltd

Thomas, V. and Dixon, A. (2012) *Improving Safety in Maternity Services: A toolkit for teams.* London: Kings Fund. Online: http://www.kingsfund.org.uk/publications/ improving-safety-maternity-services Accessed 20 July 2014

Towler, J. and Bramall, J. (1986) *Midwives in History and Society.* Beckenham: Croom Helm

Walsh, D. (2007) A birth centre's encounters with discourses of childbirth: How resistance led to innovation. *Sociology of Health and Illness* Volume 29 No. 2, pp. 216–32

West, M. A., Dawson, J. F., Admasachew, L. and Topakas, A. (2011) *NHS Staff Management and Health Service Quality: Results from the NHS staff survey and related data.* Report to the Department of Health. Online: www.gov.uk/government/publications/nhs-staff-management-and-health-service-quality Accessed 1 July 2014

Wilcox, S. (2008) *Can't supply: Can't buy: Affordability of private housing in Great Britain.* London: Hometrack

<table>
<tr><td>

3

</td><td>

Psychology and midwifery practice

Jane J. Weaver

</td></tr>
</table>

Aim

The aim of this chapter is to introduce psychology as a discipline and relate it to some of the other topics of this book. This chapter will also show the importance of psychology for midwives; not only in attempting to understand the women they care for but also for understanding themselves. It sets out to dispel some of the myths about psychology and to demonstrate how the science can broaden the way that we think about common phenomena.

Learning outcomes

By the end of this chapter the reader will be able to:

- Explain the difference between psychology and psychiatry and the appropriateness of each to the needs of the women they care for
- Reflect upon the applicability of psychological theory to situations encountered in midwifery practice
- Understand and explain the value of the main branches of psychology, and be able to apply psychological principles to both themselves and to childbearing women
- Analyse the potential contributory factors and different manifestations of perinatal mental illness
- Mount a challenge to popularist myths about pregnancy and birth, recognising the damage that these can do to women's confidence
- Deliberate upon developmental theory, applying it to the transition to motherhood and the development of new relationships in the family, as well as to bonding and attachment

---

Introduction

There are several excellent books on psychology for midwives. This chapter does not set out to provide a précis of these, although they will be referred to in places and are recommended as further reading. What this chapter aims to do is to help develop an understanding of the importance of psychology and of its value for midwives. Student midwives spend a large proportion of their training thinking about the physical aspects of pregnancy, labour and birth. This is necessary; to be a safe practitioner a midwife must have a comprehensive knowledge not only of how to manage normality but also of how to recognise and refer the woman at risk and to deal with emergencies when they arise. However, the mental health of the woman can have a profound effect on her progress through the pregnancy and childbirth journey. Even more importantly, it can impinge heavily on her self-esteem as a new mother and thus her relationship with her infant, having serious implications for her child and its development.

By 'mental health' I mean just that – mental wellbeing. It is interesting that in midwifery we so often use the term 'mental health' to mean 'mental illness'. However, we all have a level of mental health, just as we have a level of physical health. Many of us become quite vehement about the medical model of childbirth and the damage this can do to normal women experiencing a normal life event. So it is strange that when it comes to mental health we tend to adopt a similar medical, 'illness' model. But if we understand some of the principles of mental health in its broadest sense we may be able to keep the women we care for, and ourselves, healthier.

The medical model has also subtly influenced our thinking about mental health in our tendency to medicalise perceived mental health issues. For example, depression in the postnatal period is generally defined and treated as an illness (NICE, 2007). Of course many women suffering this debilitating condition feel desperate and need professional help; medical attention and medication is sometimes the best course of action. However, we do need to ask ourselves whether there may be other explanations for the way the woman feels, or at least that may be contributing to her feelings, as she may need help with these also.

To summarise, it is important that as midwives we can recognise and manage or refer mental health problems in pregnancy and the postnatal period. However, we must also identify our tendency to medicalise these conditions as well as our lack of acknowledgement of the psychological needs of the 'well woman'.

Nevertheless before we can do this we need to be clear about what psychology is and what it isn't. Therefore this chapter will begin with a definition and discussion of psychology and some of its branches. This will be followed by a brief examination of some basic psychological theories and how they can help us understand some of the behaviours we see in both ourselves and the women we care for. After this we will explore how an understanding of psychology can help us view the same phenomenon from different angles. We'll then discuss how media images of pregnancy and the postnatal period can have psychological effects on women, before considering how psychology as a discipline is evolving and examining one particular branch of psychology, developmental psychology. We will look at how it has moved beyond its traditional boundaries of bonding and child development to the study of development across the lifespan, and the relevance of this for us as midwives.

'Are you trying to analyse me?' Different psychological disciplines and perspectives and their relevance to midwives

Psychology is the scientific study of behaviour and mental processes. All psychologists begin their careers by reading for a university degree in psychology. However, there are many branches of psychology, and most involve gaining further training, qualifications or experience in the specialist area in question. Paradice (2009) discusses the lay perception that all psychologists are psychoanalysts. She recounts a common reaction to her disclosure that she is a psychologist: a look of alarm and a response along the lines of 'you're not trying to analyse me are you?'. Most of us with a psychology qualification can identify with reactions like this. However, psychoanalytic psychology is just one branch of psychology and, most would argue, a highly specialised one. Psychoanalysts are interested in the development and organisation of personality and of the human experiences and processes (including unconscious ones) that underpin these. For those interested in a psychoanalytic perspective on pregnancy and childbirth, the work of Joan Raphael-Leff will make interesting reading (for example, Raphael-Leff, 2005).

The discipline of psychology is quite separate from psychiatry, a branch of medicine dealing with the diagnosis, treatment and prevention of mental disorders. Psychiatrists begin by training to be doctors. However, one branch of psychology, clinical psychology, is concerned with the diagnosis and treatment of emotional and behavioural problems. Unsurprisingly there is some overlap between the types of conditions treated by psychiatrists and by clinical psychologists. For example, a woman with postnatal depression may be referred to a psychiatrist or a psychologist depending on her location, her specific needs and the views of the person making the referral. However, the treatments offered may be different, for example, only psychiatrists can prescribe medication.

Many clinical psychologists and psychiatrists also have an interest in the prevention of mental disorder. However, there is another branch of psychology, health psychology, which studies the psychological processes influencing and underpinning health and illness. Prevention of both physical and mental ill-health is thus also an important area of interest for this group of psychologists. For example, health psychologists research and study health compromising behaviours such as smoking, and can enable us to have a better understanding of why some women struggle to give up cigarettes while pregnant, and therefore how they can be helped (for example, Ingall and Cropley, 2010).

It can be argued that many branches of psychology have some relevance to midwives. For example, social psychologists focus on the behaviour of individuals in social situations. The theories we shall examine in the next section are from social psychology and show how it can give us insight into our own and others' actions. For instance, it can help explain why sometimes when we think we are giving a woman a choice of whether to have something or not, the woman will not perceive it as a choice at all.

Developmental psychology does what it says; it studies human development across the lifespan. Originally the emphasis, in the United Kingdom and United States, was on infant and child development but in more recent times there has been growing interest in adult development and milestones (Baltes et al., 2006). The transition to motherhood is such a milestone and one in which midwives can play an important role. The recent reduction in postnatal care is to be regretted because it is at this time that women need the help, support and confidence building that midwives are well qualified to give.

Organisational or occupational psychology seeks to understand human behaviour within the workplace. The midwifery profession and the places wherein midwives work are worthy of such study. It is important to look after, and understand, ourselves as a profession so that we can look after, and understand, the women we care for. Stress and burnout are growing problems in many workplaces (Health and Safety Executive, 2013). Moreover we must ask ourselves how we can possibly offer women control in pregnancy and childbirth if we, as midwives, do not feel in control of our work.

Educational psychology studies human learning. In a profession in which lifelong learning is essential, we need to understand the processes that will help midwives to continue to develop professionally. The theory that there are different ways of learning and that we do not all learn in the same way may enable us to enhance these processes, although more research is needed into the effectiveness of different educational interventions (Pashler et al., 2008).

The above is not a comprehensive account of the different branches of psychology. Some have not been discussed, and of those that have, the very brief summaries given here do not do justice to their depth or complexity. But the point being made in this section is a simple one: psychology is immensely useful to midwives and an understanding of some of its principles can enhance our practice in many ways. In the next section we look at some examples of these principles from social psychology.

Understanding 'normal' women like us!

In the introduction to this chapter the use of the term 'mental health' to imply mental illness was challenged. It is not just women with psychological problems that we need to understand, but the effects of the maternity care system and the challenges of pregnancy and motherhood for all women. However, even this is not spreading the psychological net wide enough. Midwives and their co-workers must also understand the psychological effects of the maternity care system on themselves.

One route into an understanding of psychology as it might affect both ourselves as staff, and the women we care for, is by examining social psychological constructs and asking their relevance to us as midwives. A psychological construct is essentially a concept that helps explain how and why people function the way they do under a given set of circumstances. Psychologists develop their constructs through empirical work and observation. Many of the classic constructs that we still refer to today were developed many years ago, although they have usually been refined over time. Paradice (2009) discusses several of these and applies them to midwifery. For example, she debates a set of psychological experiments around compliance and conformity including work by Asch (1955) and Milgram (1963). These studies show that when individuals are instructed (or asked) to do something by a person who is perceived to have authority, they are more likely to comply, even if what they are being asked to do goes against their better judgement. Also, when a person feels (or is made to feel) that they are 'swimming against the tide' (doing something that differs to the 'norm') there is a tendency to want to change, to comply with the majority, to avoid standing out or being seen as difficult. This is why it is inappropriate to gain consent to an intervention or treatment by saying to a woman 'we usually do X, is this OK?'. The woman hears, 'this is what everyone else does' and it is only a very strong woman who will then voice her disagreement. Similarly it is very stressful, in a maternity unit with a medicalised outlook, to be the midwife who stands up for normality and goes against the general flow. If you are that person in such a place of work you will understand how difficult it can feel.

Psychological constructs not only help us understand ourselves but can also sometimes point towards ways of improving our situation. Asch (1958) demonstrated that when a person gets the 'swimming against the tide' experience, it only takes one other individual to share their view to give them the confidence to stand up for what they truly think. Similarly, Milgram (1974) showed that when there is more than one voice of authority and when these voices disagree with each other, people are much more likely to follow their conscience than comply with what they are being told to do.

Because the work of Asch and Milgram is more than 40 years old it would be easy to dismiss it as dated. However such research digs deep into the workings of the human psyche and thus still has relevance today. These studies suggest that both women and midwives need allies. Women need to be told when there are alternatives to the option being recommended, and they need to feel that their view is being respected if they do not want the recommended option. Of course this process should include a full discussion of the pros and cons of each course of action. As midwives we need to gather around us a group of like-minded, enlightened midwives, or student midwives, who feel as passionate as we do about normal birth and about supporting women's choices. If you cannot find these in your own organisation (although if you look more closely you may find that like-minded people are there but are hesitant to speak out), then think seriously about joining one of the excellent support organisations for women and midwives such as the Association of Radical Midwives (ARM) or the Association for Improvements in the Maternity Services (AIMS).

Trigger

Think about your practice experiences and identify a situation where you either felt that you were swimming against the tide, or where you conceded to the views of others even though you felt they were not right. Reflect upon this situation. How did it make you feel? Why did you feel like this? Find out about the support groups available to midwives and women both locally and nationally, how they can help and how they can be contacted.

Of course, one of the most important allies for a childbearing woman can be, and should be, her midwife. Being 'with woman' is not only about being a physical presence but it is also about being a psychological support. For example, my work on control issues during labour and birth (Weaver, 1998) showed that women could feel as threatened when being given control they did not want as when they perceived themselves to be denied control. Ultimate control, for the women in my study, was being able to relinquish it and take it back again at will. Only when the midwife was able to make the woman feel supported in mind as well as in body could a close enough bond be formed for the woman to gain this level of control. And midwives could only give this level of control when they had confidence in their own practice and felt supported by their peers and colleagues.

In essence, it is impossible to be a fully rounded midwife in the true sense of the word without understanding ourselves and the women we care for.

Application to practice

Grace was finding things difficult. She was a newly qualified midwife and Debbie was almost the first woman she had cared for since she had been rotated to the delivery suite. Grace really wanted to give Debbie the best possible care, but on admission, Debbie had said that she didn't want any vaginal examinations (VEs) through her labour. Grace had reported this to the midwife in charge and had been told that VEs were important and that Grace should try to persuade Debbie to agree to them. Later that morning when, despite Grace's best efforts, Debbie's labour was progressing rather slowly, the doctor had suggested augmentation with Syntocinon. Grace had discussed this at length with Debbie, who was very unsure. She was getting really tired and yet she hadn't wanted any interventions. She had said to Grace, 'If you were me what would you do?'. Grace knew that she could not make the decision for Debbie and yet this was a choice that Debbie really did not want to make and she felt that Debbie had started to trust her . . .

Unpick the control issues in the scenario and analyse what is happening. What would you do if you were Grace?

More than one way to crack an egg: Using psychology to view a phenomenon from different angles

Until fairly recently if a woman was unhappy in the postnatal period, she was likely to be diagnosed as suffering from postnatal depression. The exceptions were when her low mood was soon after the birth and transient, in which case it would be labelled the 'blues' or if she was exhibiting psychotic behaviour when the diagnosis was likely to be puerperal psychosis. However, there has been a growing recognition that: first, not all postnatal psychological disturbance is depression; second, that problems in the postnatal period are sometimes the continuance of problems that arose in the antenatal period or are due to the type of birth the woman had; and third that postnatal depression is not necessarily different to other forms of depression and that an 'illness' explanation may not be sufficient.

Raynor and England (2010), whose excellent chapter on perinatal mental illness deserves close study, describe the term 'postnatal depression' as an outmoded and erroneous label for postnatal psychiatric disorder. They discuss a range of psychiatric disorders that may occur in the puerperium. Midwives need to be aware of all of these to enable them to recognise the woman at risk of mental illness. These include pre-existing serious mental illness: the psychotic disorders; previous psychological disorders, for example, depression, phobia and panic attacks (any of which could impinge on women's experiences of pregnancy and childbirth); emotional distress as a result of birth trauma; and medical conditions caused by, or mistaken as, psychiatric disorder.

Despite this, there is a type of postnatal depressive condition that is still frequently labelled as postnatal depression. However there is no consensus as to its aetiology, and it is likely that what we are seeing are the results of a cluster of factors that affect different women differently but that are all stamped with the one label (NICE, 2007). This is where it is helpful to look beyond the medical model of postnatal depression as an illness to also take into account some of the explanations mooted by different branches of psychology.

Postnatal depression has been studied for many years and by many different disciplines. It is deemed to be the most common medical complication of childbirth (Henshaw, 2012). Nevertheless there is considerable confusion as to what postnatal depression is and the frequency of its occurrence. Many authorities cite a prevalence of 10–15 per cent (Brown and Lumley, 2000), but some claim that it affects as many as 60 per cent of women (Halbreich and Karkun, 2006). This wide variation has been attributed to both the different methodological approaches used by researchers and to social and cultural factors (Henshaw, 2012; Ussher, 1989). However, alongside this there is a lack of consensus over the symptoms and indeed, whether the condition is a discrete type of depression or whether it is no different to clinical depression that occurs at other times (NICE, 2007). There is also wide variability in reported time of onset and duration (Henshaw, 2012). All this has led some authors to argue that postnatal depression is not a discrete entity at all (Paradice, 2009; Ussher, 1989).

Nevertheless depression during pregnancy is one of the strongest predictors of depression in the postnatal period (Robertson et al., 2004) and, despite the confusion over postnatal depression, there is no doubt that when a mother is depressed in the postnatal period this can have profound effects on her and on her family. Research has linked depression in the mother with cognitive, emotional and behavioural problems in the infant and young child (Grace et al., 2003). However, depression after childbirth also affects the woman's relationship with her partner, family and other children (Lee and Chung, 2007).

Paradice (2009) summarises the medical model of health and illness as the assumption that for every set of symptoms or diagnosis there is an underlying cause. She goes on to point out that to date there has been no causal theory of postnatal depression that fully explains all the facts. Some medical opinion has attributed postnatal depression to the rapid decline in progesterone and oestrogen levels that takes place after childbirth, effectively labelling it as an illness (Wisner et al., 2002). However, such a causal association has not been proved conclusively. Social psychologists and those that draw on social psychology for their theory (for example, Paradice, 2009 and Nicolson, 2010) point out that the list of potential postnatal depression symptoms, such as tiredness and feeling helpless, could as easily be considered a normal response to the demands of motherhood. Paradice also observes that stereotypes of motherhood, perpetuated by the media, are almost invariably positive. Thus the woman who struggles to cope with the demands of a new baby, as all women will from time to time, will be made to feel inadequate at best and despairing at worst. Unattainable role models of women who successfully juggle motherhood with a high-profile career can add to the normal woman feeling a sense of failure. Nicolson points out that postnatal depression can be brought about through guilt, anxiety and the stress from not feeling good enough as a mother, partner or professional. She has also argued that the symptoms might be argued to be normal when one considers the seismic shift in a woman's life on becoming a mother (Nicolson, 1990). She maintains that it is an inappropriate illness definition that is the problem, not the condition itself.

Feminist psychologists would agree with the above and also point out that many of the most influential psychological constructs, including those discussed earlier in this chapter, are based on studies in which all the participants were male. Thus the norm established on the basis of these studies is actually the male norm. However, it is frequently applied to both men and women. Raynor and England (2010) point out that when women's behaviour differs from that of men, it is often judged to be abnormal. Thus women are deemed to be much more prone to mental health problems, especially depression and eating disorders. In other words, if the early psychologists had studied women predominantly and seen female emotions as the norm, with their fluctuations and reactivity to life events, then quite possibly male emotional patterns would have been deemed pathological.

The important factor in this discussion on some of the different understandings of postnatal depression is to realise that there will be no 'one size fits all' cure. Many women are helped by antidepressants. Some are helped by hormone therapy. Others need counselling and support. Most need a mixture of these alongside empathy and understanding.

Trigger

Find out more about the different types of perinatal psychiatric illness and their management (for example, obtain or borrow a copy of Raynor and England's (2010) book, *Psychology for Midwives*, and read Chapter 4 on perinatal mental illness). Then ask friends and colleagues from different cultures and backgrounds their understanding of postnatal depression and how it should be treated. Are there any recurring patterns? For example, do people from cultures where family ties are tight deal with depression differently?

This section began by pointing out that midwives need to be aware of a full range of possible mental health issues that might affect the childbearing woman, to enable them to recognise the woman who is at risk of serious mental illness. However, the risk goes further than serious illness. Midwives must also recognise the place of perinatal mental illness in maternal mortality. Maternal death related to psychiatric illness may be the result of accidental overdose of addictive drugs; it may arise from medical or other causes related to psychiatric disorder, or it may be due to suicide. Suicide in pregnancy and the first postnatal year is one of the leading causes of maternal death and the latest enquiry into the causes of maternal death in the UK (CMACE, 2011) reported that since 1997 there had been no significant reduction in maternal suicide in the first six postnatal months. Nevertheless the report points out that the suicide rate amongst postnatal women is little different to the rate among women in the general population, while it is lower in the antenatal period. However, the report suggests that for women suffering from serious mental illness the suicide rate may be significantly higher. Moreover the mode of suicide is more likely to be violent in these women, for example by hanging or from multiple injuries due to jumping from a height, while women more generally tend to take their own lives by poisoning from drug overdose (Office for National Statistics, 2014).

The National Institute for Health and Care Excellence (NICE) guidelines for antenatal and postnatal mental health (NICE, 2007) point out that the routine contact with healthcare professionals that childbearing women receive in the course of their care is an opportunity to identify those who have, or who are at risk of developing, a mental disorder. Because of the very serious ramifications for the woman and her family when such disorders are missed, it is essential that midwives recognise their vital role as part of this healthcare team. Being able to only recognise physical issues with the pregnancy is to only give women half the care they deserve. An understanding of psychological issues is not optional.

Application to practice

Grace was now working in the antenatal clinic. She was becoming more confident. When she had seen Mina for a check-up in her late pregnancy she had just known that something was not right. Everything seemed fine with the pregnancy but Mina was exceptionally worried about the forthcoming birth. There was no obvious reason for this, but her birth plan was several pages long, full of minute detail. Mina was convinced that something was going to go wrong with the birth and told Grace that she couldn't sleep for worrying about it. Ignoring a colleague who had said that Mina was probably just a control freak and to not be concerned if the pregnancy was OK, Grace had made arrangements for Mina to see the psychologist who had diagnosed an anxiety state. Mina was now getting help.

Find out which psychological referral services are available at your unit. If possible make an opportunity to talk to the specialists from these services to better understand how they can help the women you care for.

The psychology and mythology of pregnancy and birth: Nappy brain and mummy tummy

Pregnancy and childbirth are life-changing events in every way. For some women motherhood will be a new and welcome role. For others the new baby is an addition to an established family. In some cases the pregnancy was unplanned and there may or may not have been acceptance by the time the baby arrives. But Sherr (1995) points out that, whatever the situation, a new baby will have a profound effect on many areas of the woman's life: her roles, employment, sexuality, finance, housing issues, lifestyle and satisfaction. Moreover Sherr observes that the literature tends to emphasise effects on the mother, but that fathers and siblings also experience upheaval. Added to this can be the media that exacerbates and intensifies the psychological effects described above. It can unsettle the new mother either by portraying motherhood as an idyllic state, or by coining pejorative terms to describe the normal experiences of postnatal women. One such term is the 'mummy tummy' or 'baby bulge' used sometimes to describe the pregnant abdomen, but also the postnatal effects of stretched abdominal muscles and pregnancy weight gain (Innes, 2013). While perfectly normal, it is often presented as an aberration, for which the Internet is full of supposed remedies, whilst newspapers seem to delight in highlighting celebrities who have regained their pre-pregnancy figures within a few weeks of the birth (for example, Reeves, 2012). For a woman struggling with the aforementioned upheavals to her life, and probably self-conscious about the changes to her body as a result of childbirth, it is easy to forget that such celebrities have means that most women can only dream of. Such resources might include money for plastic surgery or for a nanny to care for the infant while the woman meets with her personal trainer.

Another favourite media tag is the 'nappy brain'. Other terms used are 'mumnesia' and 'baby brain' (for example, Gray, 2013). Again the term seems to be equally applied both during pregnancy and in the postnatal period and refers to the perceived decline in cognitive performance that many women experience before or after birth. Research throws doubt on the existence of this condition, finding little difference between the cognitive abilities of women before, during and after pregnancy (Christensen et al., 2010). It is suggested that tiredness and emotional upheaval may contribute to the perception that the brain is working less efficiently than usual, while uncomplimentary images of the scatter-brained pregnant or new mother make women more aware of their errors than usual and thus fuel the belief that such mistakes are being made more frequently (Crawley et al., 2008).

These, and similar, images are no more helpful to women than the idealisation of motherhood. The latter presents a picture of parenthood that no woman is going to achieve, thus generating a sense of inadequacy, while the former denigrate women at a time when, because of all the changes to their lives, they are already feeling vulnerable. Some women manage to ignore them, while others find help and support with other women experiencing the same things. As described earlier, when a person feels that they are not alone in an experience, they feel stronger to deal with it. However, for the woman who is already feeling emotionally vulnerable, such as those experiencing an element of depression, such images are only likely to compound their distress.

Child and mother development

As described earlier, developmental psychology is the branch of psychology that studies development across the lifespan. Thus it can not only help us understand how the infant develops a bond with its mother and develops as a person, but also gives us insight into a woman's transition to the role of mother. As we have just seen, this transition is not made easy for women in Western cultures. As with social psychology, modern developmental theories about bonding and attachment are based on classic studies.

The terms 'bonding' and 'attachment' are often used interchangeably, although strictly speaking bonding refers to the parent's sense of connection to the child, and attachment as the child's relationship with the parent. Thus bonding is perceived to be part of the transition to motherhood for the woman. The concept of mother–baby bonding gained prominence in the late 1970s. Work by such researchers as Klaus and Kennell (1976) was based on evidence from animal studies, which showed how bonds were formed with the mother soon after birth. Klaus and Kennell suggested that there was a critical period immediately post-partum when, if a mother held her baby close and interacted with it, she was more likely to show attachment to her child. Despite deep flaws to some of these studies, the concept of bonding became enshrined in maternity unit policy. Greater effort was made to encourage mothers to hold their babies immediately after birth and most maternity units adopted policies of rooming in, whether mothers wanted it or not. Subsequent research did not always support these early theories about bonding (for example, Svejda et al., 1980).

The basic principle of reuniting mother and baby at birth is to be commended in many respects. Most mothers find this enjoyable and it promotes early breastfeeding. However, there are drawbacks when it is imposed. It denies the mother choice and, more importantly, it causes distress for mothers who cannot hold their babies immediately after birth due to general anaesthetic or to the baby needing intensive treatment in a neonatal unit. Moreover Paradice (2009) points out that it is an oversimplification to explain maternal–infant bonding in terms of a specific sensitive period after birth. Many mothers do not form an immediate bond with their baby but still go on to make excellent, caring mothers. Therefore mothers who are separated from their babies at birth need not fear that they will never be able to develop a close relationship. What is more, to emphasise mother–baby bonding to the exclusion of fathers and other family members is to limit our understanding of the complexity of human relationships.

The related concept of attachment is rooted in the work of Bowlby (1958) and has been further developed by Ainsworth (Ainsworth et al., 1978), a developmental psychologist. Attachment theory argues that, for normal social and emotional development to take place, an infant must establish a secure attachment with at least one primary caregiver. Attachment is thought to develop over the first two years of life. The concept of secure attachment was devised empirically by Ainsworth et al. (1978) in a series of experiments. These studies examined the behaviours of infants in a sequence of changing situations: the presence of a parent, of a stranger and when left entirely alone in the room. Different levels of attachment to the parent were identified.

Subsequent research has suggested that securely attached children develop more positive coping mechanisms than those with less secure levels of attachment (Oppenheim et al., 2007). However, work in this area has been criticised on several grounds: for concentrating on attachment to the mother to the exclusion of other caregivers; for the research being carried out in a highly artificial situation; for not acknowledging that children may show different behaviours depending on their current circumstances; and on ethical grounds for the stress it caused some of the children.

Bonding and attachment are, however, only part of the process of becoming a mother. As already discussed, becoming a parent has a profound effect on every aspect of a person's life. Raynor and England (2010) describe it as a time of role conflict that can also result in stress, anxiety and tension but that is, nevertheless, one of the most fulfilling and rewarding of life's experiences. Feminist psychologists such as Nicolson (1998) and Choi et al. (2005) point out that societal expectations of what a mother should and should not be and of what constitutes good and bad mothering often add to the stress and challenges of the role itself. Women not only have to relinquish their pre-childbirth state, which may have been an intrinsic part of their identity for many years, but also start to try to live up to a raft of expectations that are idealistic rather than realistic. However, fathers do not escape. Notions of what it means to be a good and a bad father also prevail and can be stressful for men (Henwood and Procter, 2003).

As healthcare professionals who support women and their families during this most important time in their lives, we must take into account the many different societal and cultural models of what constitutes a mother and a father and the related role of other family members. We must be broad minded, remembering that there are many different 'right' ways of doing things, and we must be ready to be analytical of the received opinion and empirical studies that inform our actions, because both can be flawed on occasions.

Conclusion

This chapter has introduced psychology and psychological theory, relating it to both ourselves and to the women we care for. As midwives we must be acutely aware of the needs of women and ready to react appropriately and supportively especially when things are not as they should be. This must include responding with understanding to psychological issues as well as being able to recognise physical problems. Midwives must challenge assumptions, both those made by society and those sometimes made by other professional people. To be 'with woman' is an awesome responsibility; it can help shape the rest of the woman's life. But for that very reason it is also one of the most privileged professions in the world.

References

Ainsworth MD, Blehar M, Waters E, Wall S (1978) *Patterns of Attachment: A Psychological Study of the Strange Situation.* Lawrence Erlbaum Associates: Hillsdale, New Jersey.
Asch SE (1955) Opinions and social pressure. *Scientific American* 193: 31–35.

Asch SE (1958) Effects of group pressure on the modification and distortion of judgements. In Maccoby EE, Newcomb TM Hartley EL (Eds) *Readings in Social Psychology*. Holt, Rinehart, & Winston: New York.

Baltes PB, Lindenberger U, Staudinger UM (2006) Life span theory in developmental psychology. In Damon W, Lerner RM (Eds) *Handbook of Child Psychology: Theoretical Models of Human Development*. Volume 1. 6th Edition. Wiley: Hoboken, New Jersey.

Bowlby J (1958) The nature of the child's tie to his mother. *International Journal of Psycho-Analysis* 39: 350–373.

Brown S, Lumley J (2000) Physical health problems after childbirth and maternal depression at six to seven months postpartum. *BJOG* 107(10): 1194–201.

Choi P, Henshaw C, Baker S, Tree J (2005) Supermum, superwife, supereverything: performing femininity in the transition to motherhood. *Journal of Reproductive and Infant Psychology* 23(2): 167–180.

Christensen H, Leach L, Mackinnon A (2010) Cognition in pregnancy and motherhood: Prospective cohort study. *The British Journal of Psychiatry* 196: 126–132.

CMACE (Centre for Maternal and Child Enquiries) (2011) Saving mothers' lives: Reviewing maternal deaths to make motherhood safer: 2006–2008. *BJOG* 118 (Suppl. 1), 1–203.

Crawley R, Grant S, Hinshaw K (2008) Cognitive changes in pregnancy: mild decline or societal stereotype? *Applied Cognitive Psychology* 22(8): 1142–162.

Grace SL, Evindar A, Stewart DE (2003) The effect of postpartum depression on child cognitive development and behavior: A review and critical analysis of the literature. *Archives of Women's Mental Health* 6(4): 263–274.

Gray P (2013) Decoding mystery of baby brain. Independent.ie 2 July 2013. Available at: http://www.independent.ie/lifestyle/mothers-babies/decoding-mystery-of-baby-brain-29384993.html. Accessed 22 May 2014.

Halbreich U, Karkun S (2006) Cross-cultural and social diversity of prevalence of postpartum depression and depressive symptoms. *Journal of Affective Disorders* 91: 97–111.

Health and Safety Executive (2013) Stress and psychological disorders in Great Britain 2013. Available at http://www.hse.gov.uk/statistics/causdis/stress/stress.pdf. Accessed 20 May 2014.

Henshaw C (2012) Postnatal depression. In Martin C R (Ed) *Perinatal Mental Health a Clinical Guide*. M&K Update Ltd: Keswick.

Henwood KL and Procter J (2003) The 'good father': Reading men's accounts of paternal involvement during the transition to first time fatherhood. *British Journal of Social Psychology* 42: 337–355.

Ingall G, Cropley M (2010) Exploring the barriers of quitting smoking during pregnancy: A systematic review of qualitative studies. *Women and Birth* 23(2): 45–52.

Innes H (2013) Mother-of-two who dreaded going out because of her 'mummy tummy' sheds 3st in FOUR MONTHS thanks to Oprah's diet pills. MailOnline 12 March 2013. Available at: http://www.dailymail.co.uk/health/article-2291989/I-got-rid-mummy-tummy-lost-3st-FOUR-MONTHS-thanks-raspberry-diet-pills.html. Accessed 22 May 2014.

Klaus MH, Kennell JH (1976) *Maternal-Infant Bonding*. Mosby: St Louis, Missouri.

Lee DT, Chung TK (2007) Postnatal depression: An update. Best practice and research. *Clinical Obstetrics and Gynaecology* 21(2): 183–191.

Milgram, S (1963) Behavioral study of obedience. *Journal of Abnormal and Social Psychology* 67: 371–378.

Milgram, S (1974) *Obedience to Authority: An Experimental View*. Harper and Row: New York.

NICE (National Institute for Health and Care Excellence) (2007) Antenatal and postnatal mental health: Clinical management and service guidance. Available at: http://www.nice.org.uk/nicemedia/live/11004/30431/30431.pdf. Accessed 20 May 2014.

Nicolson P (1990) Understanding postnatal depression: A mother-centred approach. *Journal of Advanced Nursing* 15(6): 689–695.

Nicolson P (1998) *Post-Natal Depression: Psychology, Science and the Transition to Motherhood*. Routledge: London.

Nicolson P (2010) What is 'psychological' about 'normal' pregnancy? *The Psychologist* 23(3): 190–193.

Office of National Statistics (2014) Suicides in the United Kingdom, 2012 Registrations. Available at: http://www.ons.gov.uk/ons/dcp171778_351100.pdf. Accessed 1 July 2014.

Oppenheim D, Koren-Karie N, Sagi-Schwartz A (2007) Emotion dialogues between mothers and children at 4.5 and 7.5 years: Relations with children's attachment at 1 year. *Child Development* 78(1): 38–52.

Paradice R (2009) *Psychology for Midwives. Current Issues in Midwifery*. Quay Books: Salisbury, Wiltshire.

Pashler H, McDaniel M, Rohrer D, Bjork R (2008) Learning styles: Concepts and evidence. *Psychological Science in the Public Interest* 9: 105–119.

Raphael-Leff J (2005) *Psychological Processes of Child Bearing*. Anna Freud Centre: London.

Raynor M, England C (2010) *Psychology for Midwives: Pregnancy, Childbirth and Puerperium*. Macgraw-Hill: Maidenhead, Berkshire.

Reeves G (2012) Yummy mummy tummy: How to get a post-baby flat stomach like J-Lo. MailOnline 7 July 2012. Available at: http://www.dailymail.co.uk/health/article-2170190/How-post-baby-flat-stomach-like-J-Lo.html. Accessed 22 May 2014.

Robertson E, Grace S, Wallington T, Stewart DE (2004) Antenatal risk factors for postpartum depression: A synthesis of recent literature. *General Hospital Psychiatry* 26: 289–295.

Sherr L (1995) *The Psychology of Pregnancy and Childbirth*. Blackwell Science: Oxford.

Svejda M J, Campos J, Emde RN (1980) Mother-infant 'bonding:' Failure to generalize. *Child Development* 51: 775–779.

Ussher (1989) *The Psychology of the Female Body*. Routledge: London.

Weaver J (1998) Choice, control and decision making in labour. In Clement S (Ed) *Psychological Perspectives on Pregnancy and Childbirth*. Churchill Livingstone: London.

Wisner KL, Parry BL, Piontek CM. (2002) Postpartum depression. *New England Journal of Medicine* 347: 194–199.

4

Anthropology and midwifery

Caroline Squire

Aim

The aim of this chapter is to consider the culture of medicine with relation to maternity care as a social system in itself. It will consider birthing in the UK in relation to dominant societal themes of technocracy and the concept of authoritative knowledge embedded within scientific and medical discourse. Cross-cultural analysis will be utilised to illustrate different ways of birthing from non-technocratic societies and a rediscovery of a social model of birth will be presented.

Learning outcomes

By the end of this chapter the reader will be able to:

1. Develop an understanding of the contribution of ethnography in presenting cross-cultural comparisons to illustrate different ways of knowing and birthing within other societies with different core values and how key findings may inform maternity care in the UK – *bringing the exotic to the familiar* (Helman, 2007)
2. Critically reflect on the contribution of ethnographic research in delineating different ways women experience childbirth and midwives practise midwifery in other similar technocratic societies and how some findings may reflect differing core values of these societies
3. Understand the five features of a social system and how these features relate to the current culture of birthing in the UK
4. Reflect on the concept of authoritative knowledge and the effects this has on experiences of women birthing in the UK as well as the effects on midwifery ways of practising within a system which values technocracy and scientific discourse

5. Appreciate other ways women can birth their babies and other models of midwifery practice that can enable midwives to be 'with woman' more effectively

6. Explore a social model of childbirth that will emphasise the imperative of acknowledging the notion of the 'expert through experience', that is, the belief in women's innate knowledge concerning how to birth their children. This will necessitate midwives to listen to women more deeply and engage with the culture in which they practise to reclaim a clearer identity

Introduction

Medical anthropology is the study of health, illness and healing across a variety of human societies (Janzen, 2002). Anthropology delves deeply into a culture using ethnography to study peoples and culture with participant observation as its key method of collecting data (Bowling, 2014). It can then present findings that are compared with other societies with differing cultural values and norms. Key themes can be discovered using cross-cultural analysis, the 'exotic can be brought to the familiar' (Helman, 2007). The development of such knowledge through cross-cultural analysis can inform the study of childbirth within the UK. The needs of care, patience and support, for example, are similar between women in childbirth from dissimilar societies and ethnographic research can provide a means by which different ways of providing such care can be shared.

The word 'medical' in medical anthropology refers not only to biomedicine but to practices in any society that occur to alleviate suffering, prevent ill health or maintain health, to include childbirth. These practices may be referred to as folk medicine or lay healing traditions. The discipline of medical anthropology can contribute to the understanding of how members of such societies make explicit their experiences of being healthy, being ill and what kind of resources they may access to maintain health or recover. It may also provide clarity in terms of the relationship between signs of suffering, ways of healing and how such experiences are made social – that is how the individual is allowed to play out her/his condition and how this is related to dominant cultural norms and values.

This chapter explores maternity care in the UK utilising theory from medical anthropology. The consideration of biomedicine as a social system will be analysed because this has been a major contribution of medical anthropology to the study of biomedicine. Furthermore, an exploration is presented of birthing in the UK in relation to dominant societal themes of technocracy and authoritative knowledge of science and medical scientific discourse. Throughout, experiences of both childbearing women and midwives are discussed within the UK and how both are affected by authoritarian structures and dominant positivist discourse. These experiences are compared and contrasted where appropriate with other societies with different dominant values with a view to a critical understanding of how these experiences relate to core societal values and whether they can contribute to women's experiences of childbirth in the UK. Finally, it is postulated that midwives need to reclaim their identity and practise 'with women' so that both midwives and women regain a sense that childbirth is a time for celebration, a life-changing rite of passage and not predominantly an event full of risk and fear.

Application to practice

'The doctor just said "Right! We need to book you in for induction for next week!!". I said that I do not want to be induced routinely and this doctor just waved a paper at me and said that new research shows that women of my age (40) need to be induced at 39 weeks because of higher rates of stillbirth. What do you do? You are just terrified that something will happen to your baby' (Katie, personal communication, November 2013).

This communication came from a woman, Katie, who was experiencing her first pregnancy. She was 38 weeks gestation. She did not smoke and was a healthy woman who took care of her diet and exercise. This was a much yearned for baby and Katie also wished to birth her baby vaginally, which she felt would be the healthiest start to her baby's life and, in any event, was how it should be. Katie subsequently felt disempowered and frustrated by what she perceived to be use of fear by the obstetrician in order to force her to conform to a system designed for a large group of women in childbirth and that appeared to diminish her as an intelligent individual. In this, Katie is far from alone with reports from countless numbers of women who have felt the maternity system to be like a conveyor belt where individual needs and wishes of women are ignored or subjugated to guidelines and protocols (Henley-Einion, 2009; Johanson et al., 2002; Kitzinger 2012). This has led in recent years to some women wishing to undergo elective caesarean sections with no clinical need because they see this as a clear way to maintain control (Arthur and Payne, 2005).

The core values of every culture are revealed in the beliefs and practices surrounding birth (Kitzinger, 2012). Anthropologists explore how behaviour around birth expresses core beliefs of a society through cross-cultural analysis. For example, in Sweden, in some maternity units on the day after giving birth, mothers and their babies are transferred from the hospital to an adjoining 'patient hotel', where they stay in 'five star' accommodation that offers every hotel amenity. A midwife clinic on every floor provides daily care for mothers and babies (Tunell, 1999 in Chalmers, 2012). The key point here is that this practice does not occur by chance; it reveals core values of equality and respect for women in Sweden so that resources are diverted to supporting postnatal women (World Economic Forum, 2013).

Trigger

What can you learn from the different ways in which women from other technocratic societies birth their children? Can you think of ways in which such birthing practices can inform the culture of birthing where you work in the UK?

Another different example of the contribution of medical anthropology to childbirth practices is a study of the experiences of Aboriginal women who give birth in their remote community in Australia (Ireland et al., 2011). The aim was to investigate the beliefs and practices of Aboriginal women who decline transfer to urban hospitals and remain in their remote community to give birth. The researchers used an ethnographic approach in which they collected birth histories and stories/narratives, observed and participated in the community for two years, made detailed field notes, trained and employed an Aboriginal co-researcher and consulted with a local reference group to ensure veracity of information gleaned. There were several key conclusions found in this study but one will be mentioned here and that was the repeated description of 'the lonely machine in Darwin'. Of course, this was the cardiotocographic (CTG) machine. They go further by describing the absence of companionship or warm human interaction; they met lots of people but felt they were being watched, often by men, rather than cared for. They were birthing outside their social norms and values, experienced distressing births and therefore made decisions not to birth outside their communities in the future.

This need for closeness and understanding is common to women all over the world; in many maternity settings this is being performed by relatives and/or trained doulas (Hunter, 2012) but, so far in the UK, there are midwifery models of working that can optimise the possibility of knowing women in terms of continuity of carer and one-to-one midwifery practice. However, both these models are under pressure in a maternity system in the UK that is hard pressed although, currently, homebirth teams are being developed in some maternity units (Walsh et al., 2014).

Application to practice

The notion of being 'with woman' is fundamental to being a midwife not only for healthy women in normal childbirth but also those women who have complications such as pre-eclampsia. Continuity of carer is a model of midwifery practice that has been implemented with positive results published (Hodnett et al., 2013). It seems that making relationships and feeling cared for is welcomed by women from all societies with differing core values.

Medical anthropologists often employ cross-cultural analysis to contribute to the understanding of interpretations and experiences of childbirth that are similar in different societies and those that may be considered aberrant. Birthing at home, for instance, may be thought of as a dangerous, selfish and deviant practice in many societies, particularly industrialised technological cultures (Cheyney et al., 2014). Furthermore, the concept of birth as a 'natural process' is problematic because birth is always framed by and within cultural norms and values and critical analysis from an anthropological perspective may bring to light the ways in which such childbirth practices are tied to dominant cultural belief systems and structures of authority (Janzen, 2002). Such critical understanding may be beneficial in creating systems of birthing and midwifery practice that may be more sensitive and health promoting not only for women in pregnancy and childbirth but also for midwives who find current ways of working challenging and often objectifying both for women and for themselves (Brodie and Leap, 2008).

Biomedicine as a cultural system

One of the most important contributions of medical anthropology to the study of health and healing in a society has been the viewing of healthcare systems as cultural systems in their own right. This will be considered now and forms the background from which the concept of authoritative knowledge in childbirth arises, which will be explored later in the chapter.

Hahn and Kleinman (1983) postulated that biomedicine should be seen as a discrete cultural system and examined five of its features as follows:

1. A distinctive domain and system of ideas, that is 'medicine'
2. A division of labour (i.e. medical specialities)
3. Corresponding roles, rules of practice and interaction and institutional settings
4. A means of 'socialisation' by which this domain and its procedures are taught and reproduced
5. An enterprise of knowledge construction (i.e. biomedical research)

Considering biomedicine or Western medicine as a cultural system in its own right is a powerful notion because it affects individuals who live and work within it as strongly as if making comparison with individuals in any given society with its own norms and values. As with entering any society, individuals, such as pregnant women, student midwives and midwives need to make sense of the values and norms of the maternity setting in the UK. The difficulty of conforming to these values and norms of a biomedical maternity setting in the UK is illustrated now with reference to the five features listed above.

A distinctive domain and system of ideas that is 'medicine'

Biomedicine, or Western or scientific medicine, is an entity in its own right. It is separate and distinct from other institutions that form part of any society such as the legal or financial institutions. It is supposed to be based on scientific principles with much of its knowledge seated within positivist discourse – that is quantifiable and reliable. But this is debatable, evidenced through different ways of working that can be found in delivery suite guidelines. For example, the guidelines for postpartum haemorrhage may be different between maternity units that are situated nearby to each other, thus challenging the positivist nature of biomedicine. The study of anatomy is another more certain example where knowledge is considered reliable and reproducible but even anatomy and its appreciation can alter with further analysis. An example of this concerns the anatomy of the breast. Some studies looking at the gross anatomy of the lactating breast found that the ductal system is comprised of fewer numbers of main ducts than previously thought. Furthermore, the ducts are compressible and do not contain large amounts of milk, the amount of fatty tissue in the breast is variable, and a proportion is situated within the glandular tissue (Geddes, 2007). Geddes further states that there had been little development in knowledge of the lactating breast since Sir Astley Cooper performed detailed dissections of lactating breasts more than 160 years ago.

From the examples above, it can be seen that scientific knowledge is often based on facts that have been taken for granted (Murphy-Lawless, 2012) because of dominance over midwives and passivity of women (Fahy, 2002). Knowledge that is considered as authoritative and certain by obstetricians may well not be (Davis-Floyd and Sargent, 1997); the widespread assumption that information gleaned through randomised controlled trials with large numbers of participants can be applied to individuals is not true and objectifies women. It is postulated that the development of different ways of knowing through research by midwives using ethnographic methodology to listen to women and hear their stories may enrich knowledge concerning individual women, subjectify them and air their voices (Olafsdottir and Kirkham, 2009).

Trigger

How do you think midwifery knowledge differs from obstetric knowledge? What examples can you think of where knowledge arisen from midwifery research has had a clear impact on the ways in which you practise? How will you take this forward?

A division of labour

Working within a maternity unit is hierarchical, with divisions of labour as in any society. Midwives have historically had much control over childbirth provision until midwifery services were transferred from the district to the maternity units within National Health Service (NHS) hospitals in the 1960s and 1970s following unsubstantiated but key government reports such as the Cranbrook report (Ministry of Health, 1959) and Peel report (Department of Health and Social Security, 1970). Women now birthed their babies away from the more private domain of small district maternity units or their homes to the very public domain of the maternity unit within an NHS institution. This change in childbirth provision coincided with the birth of modern, scientific obstetrics as a speciality of Western medicine – effectively, childbirth was now a medical event rather than a social one and a redefinition of a human event to a medical problem (Henley-Einion, 2009). Midwives lost much independence in their practice during this time and now were working within a patriarchal culture in which the superiority of scientific obstetric knowledge was dominant. This dominance of medical knowledge carries with it rewards and punishments (Foucault, 1979) for both midwives and women. Midwives who wish to work outside this prevailing discourse may be shunned, criticised or suffer what Brodie and Leap (2008: 153) term 'horizontal violence'. Women in childbirth, such as Katie, may be punished through fear – the obstetrician inferred that her unborn baby might die if she refused induction of labour (see Application to practice box above).

Currently it is argued that a pervading discourse of risk dominates current technological societies at a time of unprecedented prosperity (Walsh et al., 2008). This fear of adverse events has led to a burgeoning industry in insurance (Zwecker et al., 2011) and has translated into a litigious culture of maternity care in the UK (Furedi and Bristow, 2012). It is argued that the dependence on guidelines and reliance on positivist discourse for the production of scientific obstetric knowledge has diminished the value of some midwifery knowledge that does not conform to this paradigm (Davis-Floyd and Mather, 2002; MacVane, 2013), thereby reducing the credibility of the notion of autonomous midwifery practice.

Corresponding roles, rules of practice and interaction and institutional settings

In all societies or groups of people, there are specific expectations and ways of behaving and the same is true for working within a maternity unit. There is a real imperative to conform to the rules, regulations and ways of behaving in a modern maternity unit because to not do so renders an individual as deviant. For example, in the NHS maternity care system in the UK, many women choosing to birth at home or independent midwives who work outside this system may well be considered deviant (Cheyney et al., 2014).

Social anthropologists view groups of people working within an institution in terms of tribes and individuals within those tribes are very careful to maintain their identities usually through the use of symbols and language to denote status (Helman, 2007). Obstetricians have a clear identity and will work with stethoscopes around their necks and pagers in their pockets. Their name badges will denote their status and authority and they will employ esoteric language to communicate knowledge that women may not understand; midwives, by contrast, portray a more obscure identity often working in nurses' uniforms. The identity of being a midwife is not clear to many women who will view midwives as nurses who work with pregnant women and for obstetricians.

> ## Trigger
>
> In your practice, consider how you can make your identity as a midwife clear to women, their families and other healthcare professionals. What symbols do you use to denote your status as a healthcare professional? Do these symbols denote your identity as a midwife or another professional?

A means of 'socialisation' by which this domain and its procedures are taught and reproduced

The socialisation process within the NHS begins with a person's experiences of the NHS as they utilise technological services within and listen to the representations and stories of their parents, friends and family. The core values and beliefs of any society or group of people are expressed in the ways in which key events in a life such as birth and death are played out through ritual and ceremony (Kitzinger, 2012). In a techno-logical society such as the UK, these values stem from the use of quantifiable scientific principles based on positivist notions of cause and effect. Furthermore, economic demands drive provision and planning of maternity services with evident close rela-tionships to pharmaceutical companies and other manufacturers that stand to make profit out of the increasing rhetoric of risk prediction and surveillance such as CTG machinery (Henley-Einion, 2009; Murphy-Lawless, 2012). Time is of the essence in the technocratic model. Guidelines are bound by clock watching, vaginal examinations every four hours in established labour and so on. These core values do not pay homage to being 'with woman', waiting and listening, supporting and nurturing or of concepts of time that are fluid and seem to belong to a more natural pre-industrialised world (Becker, 2009; McCourt and Dykes, 2009).

In post-industrialisation biomedicine, the pregnant woman is viewed as incapable of childbirth without surveillance and treatment from the obstetrician (Fahy, 2008a). The metaphor also of the conveyor belt system of birth is used to powerful effect by Davis-Floyd (1987). In her ground-breaking paper entitled *The Technological Model of Birth*, Davis-Floyd portrays the basic tenets of this model to include the Cartesian doctrine of mind–body separation and the concept of the female body dependent on technology for successful reproduction. She argues that these notions are enacted and transmitted through routine obstetric procedures that serve as rituals through which the prevailing society draws upon the pregnant woman to put aside her individual belief system in order to conform to the dominant medical technological ideology. Currently, a substantial minority of women in the UK report negative experiences of childbirth as evidenced in the NHS survey 2013 where, among other complaints, women found their individual needs and concerns could be ignored or played down in an overworked system (CQC, 2013: 13).

In anthropology, a ritual is an action that is repeated and while it may not have a direct effect, it does transmit powerful social and symbolic meanings both to the individual and those around within the same cultural context. Rituals are often used in times of uncertainty such as funerals and births and are said to make sense out of chaos because they are culture specific and participants therein are comfortable with them and conform to societal expectations (Helman, 2007). Such meanings may not be understood by others in differing societies. If one accepts that biomedicine is a social system in its own right, then it is easy to understand that those actors within such institutions perform many rituals that are comprehensible to them but not to others outside, such as pregnant women.

Trigger

What aspects of your professional practice do you perform in a ritualistic manner? Why do you think you do this? How will your reflections inform your practice as a midwife?

Delivery suites are areas in maternity care that seem to many to reproduce the conveyor belt system in stark fashion and within them rituals are performed that convey strong messages of dependence on technology and the absolute necessity of such technology to produce the live baby. This message is understood by midwives as well as women in childbirth. This is the crux of the problem; the CTG is an example of a ritual that is performed commonly by many midwives despite current evidence suggesting that it should not be performed routinely (National Institute for Health and Care Excellence, 2007). In effect, it tethers a woman to the bed, limiting mobilisation and may render a woman passive and patient thus disempowering her as well as, often, the midwife her/himself. The midwife proceeds not 'with woman' but with CTG and both the woman and the midwife become inextricably immersed into this technocracy so that the birth of a baby is reliant on it. Much energy is expended by the midwife and, sometimes, by the birth partner, in interpreting fetal heart rate traces and looking to see when the next contraction will occur – the latter point may well be transmitted to the labouring woman as if she does not know. The core beliefs concern technology that controls birth and purports to make it safe, and not with support of women and their inherent abilities to birth their babies themselves. It is argued that midwives have become agents of a technological system because they have been socialised into it throughout their lives and through their training (Downe et al., 2011). The many rituals they carry out reinforce and validate their practice to the point where they are not aware of the dominant discourses that shape their decision making. Such ritualistic procedures serve to reinforce the importance of the use of technology in childbirth in a technological culture in the uncertain area of childbirth (Davis-Floyd, 2005).

An enterprise of knowledge construction

The final feature of biomedicine as postulated by Hahn and Kleinman (1983) concerns the construction of knowledge and transmission of such knowledge. This is now discussed with relation to how pregnant women source information, the carrying out of biomedical research and the concept of authoritative knowledge.

In the UK, women birth largely in a maternity system within the NHS. This system is based on Western, scientific medical principles that are positivist in nature; this means that diagnoses of conditions are usually clear and treatments prescribed will relate to the majority of those patients with such conditions. Research related to Western medicine needs to be quantifiable and measurable and the gold-standard research method is the randomised blinded controlled trial with large numbers of participants over several countries and the meta-analysis (Greenhalgh, 2010; Stewart, 2001). Of course there is nothing wrong with this research method for significant medical interventions, such as the introduction of a new drug, which need to be safe. However, this dominant discourse has presented major problems for women and for midwives over the last 50 years or so in that the production of scientific knowledge has become valorised over experiential knowledge (Lupton, 2003). One of the panel members participating in a Dephi study of midwifery knowledge represented this succinctly by stating that obstetric knowledge focuses on outcomes, midwifery knowledge provides guidance for the journey and seeks to make childbirth not just safe, but also empowering (MacVane, 2013).

The production of such knowledge, which will be called 'authoritative knowledge', is given even more credibility through the ranking of research methods in the NICE guidelines and Cochrane database, which give short shrift to content analysis, case studies, ethnographic methodology, narrative-based studies and other examples of qualitative research methods that are more experiential in nature and are more likely to represent feelings and attitudes of childbearing women and midwives. This production of knowledge creates and perpetuates the dominant discourse that childbirth is a speciality of medicine and too inherently risk laden to be otherwise.

The ways in which some women access information about childbirth and how to become mothers have changed radically in tandem with the technological revolution in the communications industry. Pregnant women will still learn from their mothers and family, parenting magazines and from their friends but they may also access the medical literature online in order to try to find out what is happening to them and the incredibly important decisions they are expected to make in the name of 'informed choice'. It seems that many women find the use of the Internet very helpful if they have access to a computer. In their study of Internet use by pregnant women, Lagan et al. (2011) found that four broad themes emerged:

- the validation of information
- empowerment
- the sharing of experiences
- assistance with decision making

These themes portray women as claiming back power in their interactions with midwives and obstetricians and the authors entreat midwives to work with women in their quest for knowledge, offer them the professional website addresses, although the information therein may well be authoritative knowledge, and to be prepared to discuss any information and queries they may have as a result.

However, to return to Katie, at the beginning of this chapter, she was adept at the use of databases and was able to access articles on induction of labour and caesarean sections with ease. She became so disheartened at seeing different obstetricians at every visit who did not want to discuss her feelings of not wanting to be induced that she felt that an elective caesarean section might be best which might 'guarantee' her a live baby. A key paper she accessed was the NICE guideline on caesarean section (National Institute for Health and Care Excellence, 2011). This guideline states that if a woman still requests a caesarean section after she has been referred to a healthcare professional with expertise in providing perinatal mental health support, then she should be offered a planned caesarean section even in the absence of clinical need. Of course Katie was traumatised at the mention that her baby might die if she did not conform to what the research apparently had 'proven'. Katie decided to 'give up' having a natural birth and attempted to discuss an elective caesarean section with another obstetrician. She did not anticipate any problems with this but, again, the obstetrician blocked her wishes by stating 'caesarean section has risks; there is a chance of the bowel being nipped, needing a hysterectomy and you might need blood transfusions'. Here, the use of fear was employed yet again to exert pressure on Katie to conform to what the obstetric system of maternity care desired. It is easier for pregnant women and midwives to conform to this authoritative knowledge to avoid conflict and, in doing so, become actively and unselfconsciously engaged with its routine production and reproduction (Jordan, 1993).

Way forward?

This chapter now presents suggestions to improve the experience of women and midwives in childbirth with the use of anthropological theory. It is proposed that:

1. Differing cultures of birthing should be supported within the NHS maternity system in the UK
2. Midwives must address the concept of professional autonomy more closely, which will include a clearer identity
3. The production of midwifery knowledge must provide guidance for working *with* pregnant women and seek to make childbirth not just safe, but also empowering not only for women in childbirth but for midwives themselves

In her groundbreaking book, *Birth in Four Cultures*, Jordan (1993) presents her findings from a cross-cultural comparison of birthing cultures in Sweden and the USA, which form part of a biomedical birthing culture, Holland, which has the highest homebirth rate of industrialised countries, and Mayan birthing culture from Yucatan. She presents a biosocial framework in that the biological is common to all women but the social is very different and culture specific. From her use of participant observation research methods, she reveals detailed information and postulates that each of the differing birthing systems has merit, which can be fed into the other to improve the experiences of such different women. Chalmers (2012) published her research that examined ten surveys of women's reports of their labour and birth in seven countries spanning North America and Western and Eastern Europe. She also advocates the sharing of knowledge and practices surrounding childbirth but the main point of both authors is that the social model of childbirth should not be subsumed within scientific paradigms and this could lead to more woman-centred and empowering midwifery practice that would benefit women and midwives alike. This knowledge should be shared globally and the challenge for midwives is to be able to access and implement such innovative practices in the UK, which requires not accepting the so-called authoritative knowledge of Western obstetrics. Currently, there are many schemes that promote midwifery practice such as home birth teams, case loading midwifery practice and many others. All of these need to be developed but often they contain guidelines that have not been written by midwives. Once more, obstetricians set the scene and create the culture within which midwives work and women experience. Midwives need to have a clearer identity and create their own culture of childbirth within which women are supported and their 'expertness' acknowledged (Kitzinger, 2005).

It seems that midwives still view autonomy as an essential construct of their professional ideology (MacVane, 2013) but it is hard to support this when one looks at the lack of independence midwives have in their practice and their lack of visibility in that the general public are likely to view midwives as nurses working within a medical system. Many midwives appear to move between technical and humanistic models of care (Davis-Floyd, 2005) and value scientific knowledge, using it as a way of engaging with obstetricians to underpin collaborative practice. The problem is that obstetricians rarely engage with midwifery knowledge; theirs is the knowledge that counts and is authoritative (Downe and McCourt, 2008). The challenge for midwives in the future is to value the knowledge that comes from themselves. Midwives need to continue to publish midwifery research that may be qualitative in nature and represent the nuances and artistry that can articulate midwifery practice.

At the same time, the identity of the midwife needs to be clarified in the eyes of the childbearing population. This is more easily done if midwives orchestrate the birthing environment more visibly and present themselves more clearly as midwives and not any other profession. There are arguments for and against the separation of low-risk and high-risk women and they often feed into the risk prediction and management rhetoric; however, it does mean that midwives can be the lead professional with low- to medium-risk women. The important point here is that the midwives control the high- or low-risk criteria and set the scene. Of course there are many examples of innovative midwifery practice such as homebirth teams, one-to-one midwifery practice and so on. These need to be clearly visible throughout the UK and not patchy provisions. Midwives must continue to create midwifery knowledge through the data made available from such practices. Furthermore, student midwives would be exposed to a different cultural system of childbirth where a different knowledge is created that is midwifery and woman centred and rituals used would portray nurturing, supporting and waiting; these students would register with a clearer worldview of other ways of empowering women as they birth their children.

Conclusion

When women birth their children, they remember their experiences of what happened for the rest of their lives. It is important that women have positive memories to strengthen them in their roles as mothers and not to have memories that are negative that may worsen over time (Waldenstrom, 2009). Medical domination of midwifery and birth is being challenged (Fahy, 2008a) and it is postulated in this chapter that to believe in midwifery as an autonomous profession, the identity of midwives must be reclaimed in the UK so that midwives can be more in control of the culture in which they practise and women birth. To do this, midwives need to continue developing midwifery knowledge that acknowledges the primacy of women and their stories, that is informed by other ways of knowing such as intuition and knowledge that is grounded in experience from, for example, previous births (Kitzinger, 2012). Such knowledge may be drawn from other societies that may be technocratic and other societies that have very different core values; medical anthropological study using ethnographic methods of research will continue to make a significant contribution in this field.

References

Arthur D, Payne D. (2005) Maternal request for elective caesarean section. *New Zealand College of Midwives Journal* 33: 15–18

Becker G. (2009) Management of time in Aboriginal and northern midwifery settings. In Christine McCourt (ed.) *Childbirth, Midwifery and Concepts of Time*. Berghahn Books: Oxford

Bowling A. (2014) *Research Methods in Health: Investigating health and social services*. 4th edition. Open University Press: Maidenhead

Britton C. (2009) Breastfeeding: A natural phenomenon or a cultural construct? In Squire C. (ed.) *The Social Context of Birth*. 2nd edition. Radcliffe Publishing Ltd: Oxford

Brodie P, Leap N. (2008) From ideal to real: The interface between birth territory and the maternity service organization. In Fahy K, Foureur M, Hastie C. *Birth Territory and Midwifery Guardianship*. Books for Midwives: London

Clews C. (2013) Normal birth and its meaning. *Evidence Based Midwifery*. March: 11(1) https://www.rcm.org.uk/content/normal-birth-and-its-meaning-a-discussion-paper (accessed 2 June 2014)

Chalmers B. (2012) Childbirth across Cultures: Research and Practice. *Birth* 39/4: 276–280

Cheyney M, Burcher P, Vedam S. (2014) A Crusade against homebirth. *Birth* 41/1: 1–4

CQC (Care Quality Commission) (2013) *National Findings from the 2013 Survey of Women's Experiences of Maternity Care*. www.nhssurveys.org/Filestore/MAT13/MAT13_maternity_report_for_publication.pdf (accessed 24 November 2014)

Davis-Floyd R. (1987) The technological model of birth. *Journal of American Folklore* 100: 479–495

Davis-Floyd R. (2005) Daughter of time: The post-modern midwife. *MIDIRS Midwifery Digest* 15/1: 32–39

Davis-Floyd R, Mather F (2002) The technocratic, humanistic, and holistic paradigms of childbirth. *MIDIRS Midwifery Digest* 12: 500–506

Davis-Floyd R, Sargent C. (eds) (1997) *Childbirth and Authoritative Knowledge: Cross-cultural perspectives*. University of California Press: London

Department of Health and Social Security (1970) *Domiciliary Midwifery, and Maternity Bed Needs: Report of the Sub-Committee (Chair Sir John Peel)*. HMSO: London

Downe S, McCourt C. (2008) From being to becoming: Reconstructing childbirth knowledges. In Downe S. (ed.) *Normal Childbirth: Evidence and Debate*. 2nd edition. Churchill Livingstone Elsevier: London

Downe S, Byrom S, Simpson L. (2011) *Essential Midwifery Practice: Expertise, Leadership and Collaboration*. Wiley-Blackwell: Chichester

Fahy K (2002) Reflecting on practice to theorise empowerment for women: Using Foucault's concepts. *Australian Journal of Midwifery* 15/1: 5 –13.

Fahy K (2008a) Power and the social construction of birth territory. In Fahy K, Foureur M, Hastie C. (Eds) *Birth Territory and Midwifery Guardianship: Theory for Practice, Education and Research*. Books for Midwives. Butterworth Heinemann Elsevier: London

Fahy K, Foureur M, Hastie C. (Eds) (2008b) *Birth Territory and Midwifery Guardianship: Theory for Practice, Education and Research*. Books for Midwives. Butterworth Heinemann Elsevier: London

Foucault M. (1979) *Discipline and Punish*. Penguin: Harmondsworth

Furedi F, Bristow J. (2012) *The Social Cost of Litigation*. Centre for Policy Studies IMS Ltd: Chichester

Geddes D. (2007) Inside the lactating breast: The latest anatomy research. *Journal of Midwifery and Women's Health* 52/6: 556–563

Greenhalgh T. (2010) *How to Read a Paper: The basics of evidenced based medicine*. 4th edition. Wiley-Blackwell BMJ Books: Oxford

Hahn R, Kleinman A. (1983) Biomedicine and anthropology. *Ann. Rev. Anthropology* 12: 305–333

Helman C. (2007) *Culture, Health and Illness*. 5th edition. Hodder Arnold: London

Henley-Einion A. (2009) The medicalisation of childbirth. In Squire C. (ed.) *The Social Context of Birth*. 2nd edition. Radcliffe Publishing Ltd: Oxford

Hodnett ED, Gates S, Hofmeyr GJ, Sakala C. (2013) *Continuous Support for Women during Childbirth (Review)*. The Cochrane Collaboration. The Cochrane Library. Issue 7. John Wiley & Sons Ltd: Oxford

Hunter C. (2012) Intimate space within institutionalized birth: Women's experiences birthing with doulas. *Anthropology & Medicine* 19/3: 315–326

Ireland S, Wulili Narjic C, Belton S, Kildea S. (2011) *Niyith Nniyith Watmam* (the quiet story): Exploring the experiences of Aboriginal women who give birth in their remote community. *Midwifery* 27: 634–641

Janzen, JM (2002) *The Social Fabric of Health: An Introduction to Medical Anthropology*. McGraw Hill: London

Johanson R, Newburn M, Macfarlane A. (2002) Has medicalisation of childbirth gone too far? *British Medical Journal* 324: 892–895

Jordan B. (1993) Authoritative knowledge. In Jordan B. (ed.) *Birth in Four cultures*. 4th edition. Waveland Press Inc. USA

Kitzinger S. (2005) *The Politics of Birth*. Elsevier: London

Kitzinger S. (2012) Rediscovering the social model of childbirth. *Birth* 39/4: 301–304

Lagan BM, Sinclair M, Kernohan WG. (2011) What is the impact of the Internet on decision-making in pregnancy? A Global study. *Birth* 38/4: 336–345

Laryea M. (1998) In search of childbirth knowledge. *Health Care for Women International* 19: 565–574

Lundgren I. (2010) Swedish women's experiences of doula support during childbirth. *Midwifery* 26: 173–180

Lupton D. (2003) *Medicine as Culture*. 2nd edition. Sage Publications: London

Mark A. (2007) Consider social anthropology. *British Medical Journal* 335/7612: 172

Martin GP, Leslie M, Minion J, Willars J, Dixon-Woods M. (2013) Between surveillance and subjectification: Professionals and the governance of quality and patient safety in English hospitals. *Social Science & Medicine* 99: 80–88

MacVane F. (2013) Is midwifery knowledge a relevant construct in contemporary practice? A report on an international Delphi survey. *Essentially MIDIRS* 4/5: 32–38

McCourt C. (ed.) (2009) *Childbirth, Midwifery and Concepts of Time*. Berghahn Books: Oxford

McCourt C, Dykes F. (2009) Time and childbirth in historical perspective. In McCourt C (ed.) *Childbirth, Midwifery and Concepts of Time*. Berghahn Books: Oxford

Mead M (2010) Unpicking the rhetoric of midwifery practice. In Spiby H, Munro J (eds) *Evidence Based Midwifery: Applications in context*. Wiley-Blackwell: Chichester

Ministry of Health (1959) *Report of the Maternity Services Committee (Cranbrook Report)*. HMSO: London

Murphy-Lawless J. (2012) Midwifery and obstetric knowledge: Thinking deeply about birth. *Essentially Midirs* 3/8: 17–22

National Institute for Health and Care Excellence (2007) *Intrapartum Care: Care of healthy women and their babies during childbirth*. CG55. NICE: London

National Institute for Health and Care Excellence (2011) *Caesarean section. Clinical guideline CG132*. RCOG: London (accessed: 27.5.14)

Olafsdottir O A, Kirkham M. (2009) Narrative time: Stories, childbirth and midwifery. In McCourt C. (ed.) *Childbirth, Midwifery and Concepts of Time*. Berghahn Books: Oxford

Sinclair M. (2013) Pregnancy: The 'Z generation': Digital mothers and their infants. *Evidenced Based Midwifery*. March Issue 2: Editorial

Squire C. (2009) Women and society. In Squire C. (ed.) *The Social Context of Birth*. 2nd edition. Radcliffe Publishing Ltd: Oxford

Stevens J, Dahlen H, Peters K, Jackson D. (2011) Midwives' and Doulas' perspectives of the role of the doula in Australia: A qualitative study. *Midwifery* 27: 509–516

Stewart M. (2001) Whose evidence counts? An exploration of health professionals' perceptions of evidence-based practice, focusing on the maternity services. *Midwifery* 17/4: 279–288.

Waldenstrom U. (2009) A longitudinal study of women's memory of labour pain-from 2 months to 5 years after the birth. *BJOG: An International Journal of Obstetrics & Gynaecology* 116/4: 577–583

Walsh D, El-Nemer AMR, Downe S. (2008) Rethinking risk and safety in maternity care. In Downe S. (ed.) *Normal Childbirth: Evidence and Debate*. 2nd edition. Churchill Livingstone Elsevier: London

Walsh D, Common L, Noble S (2014) Redressing the balance. *Midwives Magazine* 5: 42–43

Winson N. (2009) Transition to motherhood. In Squire C. (ed.) *The Social Context of Birth*. 2nd edition. Radcliffe Publishing Ltd: Oxford

World Economic Forum (2013) *The Global Gender Gap Report*. World Economic Forum: Geneva

Zwecker P, Azoulay L, Abenhaim H. (2011) Effect of fear of litigation on obstetric care: a Nationwide analysis on obstetric practice. *American Journal of Perinatology* 28/4: 277–284

5 Conformity and conflict in maternity services

Christine Grabowska

Aim

The aim of this chapter is to help the reader develop awareness of some of the behaviours that exist in maternity services as a result of contextual beliefs. The reader, as a result of appraising this chapter will be able to make an informed choice about their personal management of women within the maternity services; and reflect on their own service provision as a practitioner.

Learning outcomes

By the end of the chapter the reader will be able to:

1. Recognise behaviours within the maternity services that define conformity
2. Consider their own role and what part they are playing in conflict or maintaining the status quo
3. Question the possibility of changing their own behaviours
4. Evaluate their own actions in practice as a result of conflict
5. Wonder at the value of their own role and the possibilities of changing society to be a better place
6. Develop an action plan that will promote a birthing atmosphere of love

---

Introduction

The chapter questions the cultural norm of current-day labour ward practices and how women's expectations are formed. It will show through sociological theory how and why women and midwives conform to the guidelines and to the group with the greatest self-esteem and power. It will demonstrate that the cultural norm does not support nature, the mother, baby or the promotion of health. The chapter illustrates that people are brain-washed to support material gain, not only for the individual but for corporations and how this way of being reduces the presence of love and detracts from women's and midwives' individual creativity and purpose. The chapter will take you through the influences that accomplish indoctrination of the individual so that by the time some women and midwives get to the labour ward they have a belief system that supports the economy rather than their original purpose. The chapter is divided into two parts. Sociological theory is initially used to explain the conditions that create conformity by the manipulation of power. The consequences of following labour ward routines are then explored. The chapter considers simple physiology and the conditions that would enhance women's biology and mothering abilities. It then deliberates the powerful influences that are capable of manipulating people into prioritising the capitalist ethic and ends on a sombre note, viewing the potential life for a child born into an atmosphere of love. The sociological theory uses some references that are seminal and therefore will be old. The baby is referred to as 'she' throughout.

What is conformity?

Conformity is the structured, orderly and predictable routine that individuals follow as the norm. It is also a 'strategic behaviour aimed at gaining (re)acceptance' (Heerdink, 2013, p. 262). Conformity therefore has two meanings: on the one hand it makes people feel certain and on the other the behaviour is used in order to belong to a favoured group of people. This does not mean that everyone actually wants to conform to the favoured group values but they fear the consequences of not doing so.

Trigger

Compare and jot down any similarities/differences between the need to conform within gangs, cults or religious groups with those of midwives working within an institution such as the labour ward.

Merton and Nisbet (1961) define a non-conformist person as someone who wants to change accepted opinion by openly announcing their disagreement. Furthermore non-conformists are willing to challenge the accepted though covert norms. Confrontation with convention, as a form of 'expressive deviancy' has to be followed through in order to enable the majority to hold higher values (Dahlen, 2010). The majority often deal with the discomfort by labelling the deviant (the woman or midwife) and putting them to one side; by doing so they will have restored certainty and reduced dissonance. Uncertainty and diversity are seen as the natural enemies of order.

People react in different ways when they are uncertain or their beliefs are being destabilised (cognitive dissonance) – the majority will follow the path of least resistance. This sometimes can be seen in the labour wards where midwives can limit their role to working as an obstetric nurse. Obstetric nurses generally follow guidelines while depending on doctors to take the lead role in decision making regarding a plan of care. Obstetric nurses then cannot act autonomously, reducing their ability to be the woman's advocate. The behaviour is out of line with the full role of the midwife (NMC, 2012). There are a few reasons why midwives shy away from their full role. Midwives can choose the path of least resistance by conforming to the opinions of the doctors (or those with the greater power) in order to reduce their stress. Some of the midwives will act out the ritual of the routine, and call a doctor with little thought and no questioning. Other midwives will think and perform in an underhand (or innovative) way where they appear to be acting within the confines of the accepted norms and in doing so be the woman's advocate (Stewart, 2005). A few midwives choose to retreat from obstetric practice to birth centres or to independent practice, in order to act out their full role and reduce their dissonance. It is only a minority of midwives who will have the courage to rebel and are commonly known as 'the trouble makers' (Merton, 1957). These midwives stand out and stand up for the rights of midwives and women. They are the 'moral frontiersmen' (Erikson, 1966) and aim to change practice based on good evidence, kindness and compassion.

Application to practice

A woman who has had ruptured membranes for two days is requesting the use of water for labour and birth. She is apyrexial and on examination no abnormality is detected. The guidelines indicate acceleration of labour and to enter her into a high-risk category to fulfil Maternity Improvements (formerly the clinical negligence scheme for trusts) requirement to avert litigation. Consider the actions of the 'moral frontiersman' midwife?

Let us consider the midwife's choices. First, the tradition of obeying through custom and practice – 'this is the way we've always done it'. Any new evidence to supersede out-dated practices will largely be ignored in this scenario. Therefore the midwife will not consider this option. Second, the charismatic leader legitimises a practice, such as a consultant midwife or a doctor giving an order 'because I say so'. People with lower self-esteem commonly obey people with higher self-esteem and assume that they have a higher level of knowledge or experience that qualifies their opinion. If the midwife has a good level of self-esteem she could consider this option and use it to educate others. Third, conformity comes from and through rational knowledge, where the rules appear reasonable and therefore would have legal tender. Guidelines are written from evidence that is approved by a 'senior' group of 'experts'. It is through this third option that the bureaucracy of the National Health Service (NHS) is maintained. Routine practice is created from this set of 'rules' and it is in direct conflict with individual choice.

All organisations, including the NHS, have groups of social rules in order to preserve the social order such as to act hurriedly and ready for a calamity. Compare this to walking into a birth centre where the social rules expect the midwife to be thoughtful, quiet and respectful of the environment. People maintain the social order because they believe the rules are moral; that is they have a conviction that the behaviours are good. The social order provides security for everyone who works within this framework in that they believe they have certainty. Labour wards are constructed in the face of potential chaos (an emergency can happen at any time (Boyle, 2011)). In order to have certainty, guidelines are produced and the midwives and doctors practice emergency skills drills that require a good memory (Boyle, 2013; Thomas and Dixon, 2012), rather than an ability to make reasoned decisions. Labour wards delineate the risks of disease and childbirth in order to fulfil the requirements of Maternity Improvements, with a view to reducing the NHS trust litigation costs (Nair and Chandraharan, 2010). Working within an atmosphere where the notion that something could go wrong increases the chances that everyone will work very closely to the rules or guidelines (Sox et al., 2013).

Social order is possible by repetition of patterns of behaviour that become a standard response to the same situation. Once a midwife works repeatedly with the same guidelines it is possible that she can reduce her work effort and at the same time the amount of decision making she formulates will decrease. Repetitions of patterns of behaviour are learnt early by a student midwife who looks for cues. She looks to her mentor and other midwives on appropriate behaviour because her need is to conform and ultimately to pass her practice assessment. Once the student becomes a midwife the guidelines are again re-enforced during her preceptorship programme and by the time the midwife is a mentor assessor herself she is role modelling the behaviour patterns her own mentors showed her (Ferguson and Barry, 2011). The midwife has times when she is pulled away from being 'with woman' because she is feeling frightened (Dahlen, 2010). Fear usually has the effect that the midwife will conform to the established guidelines and accepted norms in preference to the woman's wishes because she believes she is protecting herself.

Anyone who defies the accepted and sometimes covert norms will be labelled deviant. Midwives can now and do make up a story based on a negative judgement about the 'deviant's' character and personality. The labelled deviant is now a target to become a scapegoat. Tensions resulting from working in labour ward can now be diffused by directing conflict towards the scapegoat (MacValue, 2013). Support for the conflict can be generated by gaining collusion from work colleagues and thus begins the labelling process.

Application to practice

Consider the woman with a long birth plan. It is written in the format of what she does not want: for instance an epidural, artificial rupture of membranes, intravenous syntocinon, third stage of labour active management, vitamin K administration to her baby. She then says she wants to be left alone with her family following the birth so that the baby can be checked and weighed at a later time. What range of behaviors have you observed by midwives in response to seeing this type of birth plan?

Non-compliance by women often gets a label of 'bad patient' (Bessett, 2010, p. 370). The sanctions can either be passive (ignoring or ostracising the woman) or active (rejecting or bullying the woman into conformity); these actions exclude the individual (Heerdink et al., 2013, p. 263). Active, even subtle, pressure is brought to bear on the 'positive deviance' (Gary, 2013).

Application to practice

A woman states at booking that she does not want any screening tests, to include bloods and ultrasound. Consider the response by all the professionals who either come into contact with her or hear about her case. Will there be any pressure put upon her to conform to the accepted antenatal care pathway, even though it is in direct opposition to her wishes?

Conforming to majority opinion may reduce dissonance for some people and others will be working within an environment of uneasy peace (Merton and Nisbet, 1961) by suppressing their own opinions.

Trigger

How do you think the 'moral frontiersman' midwife would behave in response to any negative criticism of the woman, her birth plan and her wishes not to partake of screening?

Choice for the majority of people is socially constructed and control of the labour process is out of reach for both women and midwives. Women who want certainty often put their trust in medicalisation, which includes involvement in risky procedures (Hammer and Burton-Jeangros, 2013, p. 61). There is an illusion of control as routines (for instance a labour care pathway) help people to feel certain (Dahlen, 2010). Both women and midwives then feel 'safe' as if nothing can go 'wrong'. These routines will include the use of a partogram, cardiotography, observations of blood pressure, pulse and temperature, vaginal examinations and urine testing, among others. Habitual patterns can be justified because there is an acceptance of the guidelines that appear to be integrated by all staff. Meanings given to words such as 'safety' ease discomfort for both women and midwives and while they think they are 'safe' ('nothing can go wrong') this increases their acceptance of the hospital guidelines. The guidelines can now appear as valid and true.

Conformity becomes easier when personal beliefs are aligned with the guidelines. The cascade of intervention does not guarantee outcomes, yet the guidelines create an illusion of 'safety'. So much so that even doctors who choose to routinely follow the labour ward guidelines may feel 'safe' because they are protected by the General Medical Council, despite the Medical (Professional Performance) Act (1995) delineating sanctions for doctors who act with poor judgement. The Darzi report (Darzi, 2007) reiterated that the public are disillusioned into believing that 'doctor knows best'. Despite this the accepted norm is that anyone who does not want to follow the rules or women that refuse routine 'care' are in violation with a powerful and dominant group. The group with the most power will be able to create and impose their rules and sanctions on the less powerful (Menard et al., 2011). It is this hierarchical system of control that prevents midwives from acting out their full role and women accepting a poor quality of service with the illusion that they at least will be 'safe' and treated well (Kirkham, 1999).

Some midwives defer to medical dominance because they are frightened of the consequences of not doing so ('what if something goes wrong?') and women 'do as they are told' because they too are frightened and vulnerable with a great concern for the wellbeing of their babies (Kitzinger, 2005, p. 50). The NHS bureaucratic goal is to direct the midwives' and women's behaviour in the direction of conformity. If stability is to be maintained within the labour ward then the norms have to be adhered to, thus reducing flexibility for an individual woman's choice. Women are often unaware of the rules unless they have been to the antenatal classes that impose them. Classes are usually ordered with information on what to expect. Women are then indoctrinated into the ways of behaving when they enter the hospital. Midwives compensate for women's lack of knowledge by giving information and protective steering of that information. Women may think that they have free choice and midwives may label a woman as 'irrational and wrong' when in fact they are both conforming (Pronin et al., 2007, p. 595).

Deviance is contextual so if the same woman was in labour in a different setting such as a birth centre, with midwives whose practice promotes normality, she may indeed fit into the social order of the birth centre. Some women resist medicalisation and choose a place of birth to reduce intervention. Women may choose a birth centre to enhance their feeling of security, as opposed to choosing to have their baby at home because they have a 'loss of confidence in their own bodies, dependency on professionals and undue anxiety' (Hammer and Burton-Jeangros, 2013, p. 56). There is a reduction of cognitive dissonance for the midwife in a birth centre because she can act autonomously and as the woman's advocate, acting in the role to which she was educated and registered.

Scientific medicine views the body as a machine and in labour ward the body is viewed as primarily malfunctioning (Franklin, 2014). These are negative judgements that are socially constructed. Medicine focuses on the internal environment of the body and not the external environment of the woman's life. The way a woman feels physically and emotionally has a direct effect on her pregnancy and baby (Dunkel Schetter, 2011). Her body is viewed medically as separate from the woman herself. This is seen clearly when technology is used to record what the woman often knows herself. Specimens are removed from the woman's body to be scientifically analysed away from her. It is as if science does not know that the way a woman feels can directly affect her immunity, her hormones and her labour (Wadhwa et al., 2011).

Think about this: the woman initiates her maternity service provision by attending the general practitioner (GP). At that point in time she knows she is pregnant. Why then does the GP want to confirm the pregnancy by performing a pregnancy test?

The social engagement of the midwife with the woman is known to improve women's satisfaction with the maternity services as well as improve birth outcomes (Beake et al., 2013). Once a woman is labelled with an illness or disease then the focus is on the problem that is considered undesirable (Friedson, 1970b, p. 223) and her behaviour, through fear, often changes to conform to the rules.

Illness is a label that has been produced by medical science. Risk criteria and pathology are applied to the woman and what should be her decisions are being made by the doctors. Women consider they have a moral duty to conform (Parsons, 1951) to ensure the 'safety' of both themselves and their babies. Gradually over the last century some women have expected to see pregnancy as a medical, pathological event that is permanently at risk (Hammer and Burton-Jeangros, 2013). The woman receives positive regard by midwives, family and her peers if she chooses the available technology, thus re-enforcing the medical social control. Sacrifice and suffering earns women praise and sympathy (Bessett, 2010) within the social norm. Parsons (1949) makes it clear that once a woman agrees to medical social control then she will receive the assistance of an obstetric team. When the woman enters the hospital she is not merely receiving assistance, she is also subjected to medical and bureaucratic control. The woman is however tangential to labour ward staff and will conform to gain their acceptance, giving up her normal behaviour for fear of negative reprisal (Heerdink et al., 2013, p. 272).

A labouring woman who has previously stated that she does not want an epidural in labour now feels frightened by what a midwife tells her – that her labour is progressing too slowly. Twenty minutes after this interaction the midwife notes a fetal heart deceleration and wants to call the doctor. Ten minutes after this episode the woman is requesting an epidural. Consider the physiology that is causing the fetal distress. Imagine the banter between the midwives at shift handover of this woman's care.

Midwifery as a practice is being undersold and devalued (MacLellan, 2014). The labour ward norm and a signpost of positive regard is that midwives can manage many labouring women simultaneously (MacValue, 2013). This works well for the bureaucracy of the NHS, when bound by labour ward guidelines. The process though weakens women's or midwives' ability to make individualised decisions. A midwife with high self-esteem is more likely to make individualised decisions as she would not have a great need to belong to the influential group (Ferris et al., 2009). She could focus on best care for individual women, because she is unencumbered by a need to conform. A midwife with self-awareness will know if she holds different values to those of her organisation. Midwives' education teaches best practice, so if the hospital guidelines are unrealistic the midwife must make a decision on an individual basis (Gary, 2013). The midwife accepts the risk of not acting within the guidelines, acts autonomously in her decision making and preserves women's choice (Dodge, 1985). Her actions are positive deviance whereby she is the creator of knowledge while dealing with ethical and legal dilemmas. Most midwives will recognise the covert practice of the cervical lip that if recorded correctly would be written as a fully dilated cervix (Stewart, 2005). This could be seen as negative deviance and it does not promote the integrity of the midwife.

Application to practice

A woman who has an urge to push is given a 'quick vaginal examination' and the midwife discovers the woman's cervix to be fully dilated. There is a doctor's round on labour ward and they want to know if the midwife has checked the woman's cervix because they observe she is pushing. What are the actions of the 'moral frontiersman' midwife?

Conformity increases group cohesiveness by the sharing of similar norms and values (Zoghbi-Manrique-de-Lara, 2010). By recording the cervical lip the midwife conforms to the hidden agenda of her colleagues. Integration of new practices and truth telling will only happen when the guidelines are written to reflect these and on occasion penalties are enforced in order to see those changes in practice. The 'moral frontiersman' midwife is essential in bringing the truth to the fore so that guidelines reflect good practice. Change is slow when encouraged by the public who, for instance, may not know what the NHS constitution (DH, 2009) includes or the rights and standards that it contains. The public demand for positive change can be limited even though the Health and Social Care Act (DH, 2012) has addressed this. It is up to midwives to provide excellence and not wait for public demand. Positive deviance can support midwives to work effectively and produce better outcomes for women.

Human programming

The second part of this chapter will now look at human programming and why it is so important for midwives to protect the process of birthing. Midwives can work together as a team in supporting women once they understand and believe in women's innate ability to birth their babies. Midwives can begin to respect themselves when they know that their role is in maintaining women's nature and literally standing alongside by 'being with' women. Currently the erosion of the midwife's role and devolution to doctors and maternity assistants is happening because of conforming (Davis and Walker, 2013; Mander and Fleming, 2002). The chapter now looks at some of the reasons why midwives are needed by women and discusses the long-term impact midwives have not only on the family but the whole of society.

Nature and human beings have an integral programming system so that by design innate behaviours regulate life (Atzil et al., 2011). These behaviours are modulated through hormonal processes for reproduction and they also exist to ensure the baby's safety and longevity. This can be seen simply as an uncontrollable sexual urge in puberty for girls and boys that may eventually lead to the growth of a family. The baby comes into the world with the ability to tune others to her needs, through the use of all her senses. The baby does not even resemble the adult and yet she has the ability to affect every one of her mother's senses (Hales et al., 1977). Sense stimulation can be explained through animal husbandry that evolved to prevent many lambs being rejected by their mothers. The ewe licks her lamb clean following birth and this innate act will fine tune the ewe's senses to her lamb, and it becomes the primary source of attachment. The ewe thus develops her sensory perception of taste, smell, vision, hearing and feel for the lamb (Collias, 1956; Domjan, 1987). The farmer knows that he must not interfere with this process or the lamb will either smell or taste 'wrong' to the ewe and thus be rejected.

Human programming has been altered by the hormones of fear and belief in the birthing cultural norm. The human female, unlike the ewe, has the addition of logic and can often use this to rationalise her birthing experience and resulting outcomes. She does though have no understanding of the way she responds to her baby and some-times she does this with feelings of negativity following a medicalised delivery. There has been a rise in postnatal depression from 10 per cent 20 years ago to 19 per cent currently (O'Hara and McCabe, 2013). Poor maternal–infant attachment behaviours are greater if a woman has a planned epidural or caesarean section (Fenwick et al., 2012; Olza-Fernandez et al., 2014). The nature of depression is to be self-centred and thus she may reject her baby (Gunning et al., 2004; Kaplan et al., 2004). Women also have three times more morbidity following a caesarean section than a vaginal birth (Park et al., 2005).

Women having an epidural 'package deal' are more likely to suffer a cascade of intervention (intravenous fluids to control blood pressure and prevent hypotension, bladder catheterisation because of sensory loss to the detrusor muscle, electronic fetal monitoring because of an increased risk of fetal distress, immobility in order to monitor the mother and baby effectively, instrumental or operative delivery because of fetal distress and, as a result of these modes of delivery, an episiotomy or an abdominal incision). The side-effects of epidural anaesthesia result in possibly a poor mechanism of labour due to poor pelvic floor muscle tone, hypotension, hyperthermia due to vasodilation, backache at point of needle entry due to rupture of a blood vessel, nerve damage at the point of needle entry, a dural tap because the needle has proceeded beyond the dura and into the cerebro-spinal fluid and, extremely rarely, paralysis

(Gaskin, 2008). Epidural anaesthesia also interferes with an effective hormonal input from the woman that would assist in her own process of birthing (Carter, 2014). An epidural is designed to remove sensory stimulation; the birth is the very time when a woman needs all her senses to get to know and love her baby.

The hormonal input of the birthing process (prostaglandins, oxytocin, oestrogens, progesterone, corticotrophin releasing hormone, beta-endorphins) achieves the innate fine tuning of the mother's senses, thereby programming the relationship for attachment and love (Dixon et al., 2013). The hormone oxytocin is released in a pulsatile manner throughout labour, having a major role through the Ferguson reflex in the second stage of labour to enable the baby to be born. Oxytocin is the love hormone (Carter, 2014; Odent, 1999). It is released at critical times in our lives such as at orgasm, breastfeeding and birth when a huge surge of this hormone can be measured from the Ferguson reflex (Nissen et al., 1996). The Ferguson reflex is absent in women who have opted for epidural anaesthesia or in those who are having caesarean sections.

Trigger

Consider the effects of withholding mother–infant attachment on both the mother and baby by withdrawing the love hormone, oxytocin, heightened through the Ferguson reflex.

The physiology of mother–infant attachment can be understood following a natural birth by being compared to meeting a dream partner. The physiology changes to a sympathetic, autonomic nervous system response of tachycardia, perspiration and heightening of all the senses when the woman meets a partner she is attracted to, as well as meeting her new born. The baby shares the natural maternal hormonal cocktail of adrenaline and oxytocin, which she will have received via the placenta. The baby thus has dilated pupils, which attracts her to her mother. The catecholamine response that leads to dilation of pupils for both mother and baby will reduce the clarity of distant vision and increase near-sightedness. The mother concentrates on the baby's eyes initially and then her eyes wander around the baby's face taking in its structure and contours. She takes the baby's hands and unfolds her fingers and feels each one, then the baby's feet and touches each of her toes (Finigan and Davies, 2004). She strokes her baby's face while still gazing at her and as the desire takes hold she will kiss her baby, while tasting and smelling her at the same time. All the time she is hearing the noises her baby makes. She strokes her baby's arms and legs and looks at her chest and tummy as she continues to move her strokes inwards towards the centre of the baby's body and down over her back and buttocks and she needs to check for herself that she has a girl (Anderson et al., 2005). If the baby is left on her mother's skin she will move, touching her own mother, while listening to what her mother is saying. Using her own sense of smell she will find her mother's breast, tasting her mother's colostrum (Nishitani et al., 2014; Odent, 2003). This will maintain the release of maternal oxytocin and ensure that the mother literally has attached to her baby

(Carter, 2014; Nissen et al., 1996). Compare this to getting to know an attractive partner's body! Nature has now set the scene for falling in love.

Just after birth the baby will remain in a state of alertness for approximately two hours (Klaus and Kennell, 1976). This provides a window of opportunity for getting to know each other following the birth. This relationship needs to be left undisturbed, as similarly wanting to be left uninterrupted with the partner of your dreams. The relationship has developed unconsciously and as a result the mother could pick her baby out from a room full of babies. She would be able to recognise her baby's cry above all other babies' cries and not unusually she would wake identifying that her baby is hungry prior to her baby demanding a feed. It is actually the birthing experience that can ensure that the mother is attuned or programmed to her baby. The result is that as the mother continues to use her senses she will never let the baby come to any harm (Hatfield and Rapson, 2000). That is the miracle of nature!

Trigger

How can you see midwives and doctors supporting the production of the love cocktail of hormones within a peaceful, low-stimuli birthing environment?

The world we live in is chaotic and life is uncertain and this is never clearer until a baby enters a relationship. People live under the false assumption that they are organised, that their life is predictable and that they are in control. People that live their daily lives going out to work have a linear expectation that a=b and when c comes along they see it as a problem, usually reminding them that life is not under their control. This linear way of thinking is set up by society; the work place (including labour wards) keeps us feeling comfortable because it is predictable! Most mothers expecting their first child think that the linear model can then be applied to their life with a baby and thus women who have never had a child will be saying 'the baby will fit into my life'. Women could choose to learn so much about themselves and be empowered by the birth process, instead some choose to avoid labour and make the process predictable (by having a planned caesarean section or an epidural anaesthetic) because they think they will not survive the process (Levine, 2005), nor the pain and they don't want to 'fail' when birthing in front of strangers. Now that the mother feels uncertain she doesn't want to show her vulnerability (Barrett et al., 2007). She is frightened and chooses a route for labour where she feels in control with desired and expected outcomes. She reached this point in her life by conforming and being socialised by all the influences put along her life's path. Overcoming her fear enhances her self-belief, allows the presence of her true nature and thus creates her own true empowerment.

The birth industry is very profitable; it centres on hospitals to promote pharmaceuticals and machinery manufacturers' equipment. Labour wards and operating theatres are the biggest purchasers of drugs and equipment. We live in a capitalist culture where materialism is the norm (Tellis et al., 2009). Midwives, doctors and parents are surrounded by influences that will propagandise them into unconsciously believing that their lives are improved by purchasing goods and services. This belief is the basis of the capitalist ethos and may indeed conflict with the promotion of health. There are examples of capitalism at work within the NHS. For instance insurance companies benefit from malpractice and all practitioners cannot work without liability insurance (NMC, 2015). Bureaucratised medicine is dependent on technology. Obstetrics has succeeded in both therapeutic and economic expansion. Subconsciously some midwives support the economy by the use of drugs and machinery rather than being 'with woman'. That is the power of cultural indoctrination.

Cultural indoctrination and thus conformity begins when we are socialised by our parents to fit the society to which we are born (Meyer et al., 2014). The next main institution that will indoctrinate us is formal education. Every child has to follow the school curriculum and pass certain tests along the way (Django, 2012). Competition is encouraged very early with school exams and sports where children compare themselves with each other (they compare their results, their looks, their clothes, their behaviour and so on). Some children learn that life is about achieving, succeeding and meeting targets. The label 'failure' is a thing to be avoided. This sets them up for the world of work, where there will be deadlines to meet, agendas/guidelines to follow and expectations for certain behaviours. Most people accept this because they now see the reward beyond passing exams and this is often monetary gain, which again is the focus in any materialistic society.

Another influence is a peer group or friends, who will pressurise each other to look the same, think the same way, feel similar emotions and do the same as each other. These groups will be influenced by all the major institutions of that society. Furthermore, the public communications that parents, midwives and doctors have been exposed to will re-enforce these belief systems. We are influenced by advertising on all media (radio, television, marketing, magazines, news). These media often stunt a child into conformity when they see and hear images and stories of societal expectations and clear messages of 'right' and 'wrong'. Gaining and spending money is prioritised through these media (Tellis et al., 2009).

The next major influence to continue the indoctrination process will be the workplace. Here people will learn to behave in ways that are expected from them in order to fit in. The parent, midwife or doctor have been moulded and are losing sight of who they once were and they are adapting the work persona to mean it is their real self. Most of all they will, at this time in their life, be focused on knowing all the things they cannot do, as often revealed to them by their parents and at school, and so they will be insecure. This often prevents them from ever trying to know their own true worth because they will want to be employed, with a salary, as a form of security. They will narrow their focus even more than at school, as the job becomes specialised and this will serve to confirm the limitations that they have come to believe about themselves.

There are other media that will influence the child such as religious groups, party politics or membership of clubs or societies. It is very rare indeed for midwives, doctors and parents to withstand all of these pressures and to be able to stand out and be different. It would be easy to blame the individual for their choices. Most people have little or no awareness of making any decisions as they mindlessly follow the cultural belief.

The baby is short changed within our cultural norm. Without the exquisite hormonal cocktail that is naturally produced at birth where the mother begins loving and attaching to her baby, she instead will have to start learning to love her baby over a period of time.

Trigger

What kind of world do you want for your children?

Imagine the effects of programming children into a life with the continuous presence of love that ultimately would have a dramatic and far-reaching effect on the whole planet – one in which everyone cares for each other and their environment, one in which we have respect for individuals and their own needs, one in which we can have honest and open communication because it can only be coming from a place of love. A child growing up in an environment that supports who they are will enrich everyone. Let us continue by nurturing and prioritising the growth of love in our labour wards and then enhancing its spread, whereby it is the norm within individual families. Consequently a child grows up with confidence and does not have to look outside of herself for approval. She knows her own beauty as she becomes an adult; she doesn't need endorsement by others and nor does she aspire to copy images on the television or magazines and thus want to change her body with surgery, make-up or clothes. She is self-assured because she knows that she is perfect the way she is. She will grow up to accept herself and other human beings; she will congratulate individuals for their achievements and be happy for them because she is not trying to compete with them. She truly is free as she develops her own spirit, and delights when others take joy from what she can share with them. It is the greatest gift a midwife can bestow when she is 'with woman' to ensure the birth of a better world.

Conclusion

This chapter considered the sociology of conformity and how it is reckless in the labour ward, withdrawing women's choice for a natural birth, while putting great pressures on starting a new family by not having her own hormonal cocktail to support the immediate growth of love. It also mentioned the impact that the resulting negative emotional effect could have on women. It considered the burdens that envelope the midwife who works consciously or unconsciously to conform and the sequelae of her own choices. Subsequently the chapter went onto endorse a birth environment of love for the emerging baby, which would then develop within the family and she would grow to share love with others. The chapter makes the case for the promotion of love through leaving women undisturbed throughout labour so that they will engender their own power for motherhood.

References

Anderson, G.C., Moore, E., Hepworth, J., Bergman, N. (2005) Early skin-to-skin contact for mothers and their healthy newborn infants. *The Cochrane Library* Oxford (3) ID # CD003519

Atzil, S., Hendler, T., Feldman, R. (2011) Specifying the neurobiological basis of human attachment: Brain, hormones and behaviour in synchronous and intrusive mothers. *Neuropsychopharmacology* 36: 2603–2615. http://www.nature.com/npp/journal/v36/n13/pdf/npp2011172a.pdf Accessed 15 August 2014

Barrett, L.F., Mesquita, B., Ochsner, K.N., Gross, J.J. (2007) The experience of emotion. *Annual Review of Psychology* 58: 373–403

Beake, S., Acosta, L., Cooke, P., McCourt, C. (2013) Caseload midwifery in a multi-ethnic community: The women's experiences. *Midwifery* 29 (8): 996–1002

Bessett, D. (2010) Negotiating normalization: The perils of producing pregnancy symptoms in prenatal care. *Social Science & Medicine* 71: 370–377

Boyle, M. (2011) *Emergencies Around Childbirth*. London: Radcliffe Publishing

Boyle, S. (2013) Women's views on partnership working with midwives during pregnancy and childbirth. DH Res University of Hertfordshire *http://uhra.herts.ac.uk/bitstream/handle/2299/10919/05111975%20Boyle%20Salle%20-%20final%20DHRes%20submission.pdf?sequence=1* Accessed 26 June 2014

Carter, S.C. (2014) Oxytocin pathways and the evolution of human behaviour. *Annual Review of Psychology* 65: 17–39

Collias, N.E. (1956) The analysis of socialisation of sheep & goats. *Ecology* 37: 228–239

Dahlen (2010) Undone by fear? Deluded by trust? *Midwifery* 26 (2): 156–162

Darzi, A. (2007) *Our National Health Service, Our future National Health Service Next Stage Review: Interim report*. London: Department of Health www.dh.gov.uk

Davis, D., Walker, K. (2013) Towards an 'optics of power': Technologies of surveillance and discipline and case-loading midwifery practice in New Zealand. *Gender, Place & Culture: A Journal of feminist Geography* 20 (5): 597–612

DH (Department of Health) (2009) *The NHS Constitution*. London: Department of Health

DH (2012) *The Health and Social Care Act*. London: Department of Health

Dixon, L., Skinner, J., Foureur, M. (2013) The emotional and hormonal pathways of labour and birth: Integrating mind, body and behaviour. *New Zealand College of Midwives Journal* 48: 15–23 http://dx.doi.org/10.12784/nzcomjnl48.2013.2.15-23 accessed 15 August, 2014

Django, P. (2012) Culturally sustaining pedagogy. *Educational Researcher* 41 (3): 93–97

Dodge, D. L. (1985) The over-negativised conceptualization of deviance: A programmatic exploration. *Deviant Behaviour* 6 (1): 17–37

Domjan, M. (1987) Animal learning comes of age. *American Psychologist* 42 (6): 556–564

Dunkel Schetter, C. (2011) Psychological science on pregnancy: Stress processes, biopsychosocial models and emerging research issues. *Annual Review of Psychology* 62: 531–558

Erikson, K.T. (1966) *Wayward Puritans*. New York: John Wiley & Sons Inc.

Fenwick, J., Hauck, Y., Schmeid, V., Dhaliwal, S., Butt, J. (2012) Association between mode of birth and self-reported maternal physical and psychological health problems at 10 weeks postpartum. *International Journal of Childbirth* 2 (2): 115–125

Ferguson, M., Barry, B. O. (2011) I know what you did: The effects of interpersonal deviance on bystanders. *Journal of Occupational Health Psychology* 16 (1): 80–94

Ferris, D. L., Brown, D.J., Lian, H., Keeping, L.M. (2009) When does self-esteem relate to deviant behaviour? The role of contingencies of self-worth. *Journal of Applied Psychology* 94 (5): 1345–1353

Finigan, V., Davies, S. (2004) 'I just wanted to love, hold him forever': Women's lived experience of skin-to-skin contact with their baby immediately after birth. *Evidence based midwifery* 2 (2): 59–65

Franklin, J. (2014) A mother's paradox: Choosing a birthing method in the 21st century. *Pitzer Senior Theses* Paper 57. http://scholarship.claremont.edu/pitzer_theses/57 Accessed 14 August 2014

Freidson, E. (1970a) *Professional Dominance*. Chicago: Atherton Press

Freidson, E. (1970b) *The Profession of Medicine*. New York: Dodd, Mead and Co.

Gary, J.C. (2013) Exploring the concept and use of positive deviance in nursing: 'Responsible subversion' and why accurate documentation matters. *American Journal of Nursing online.com* 113 (8): 26–34

Gaskin, I.M. (2008) *Ina May's Guide to Childbirth*. New York: Vermilion

Gunning, M., Conroy, S, Valoriani, V. Figueiredo, B., Kammerer, M.H., Muzik, M., Glatigny-Dallay, E., Murray, L. (2004) Measurement of mother–infant interactions and the home environment in a European setting. *The British Journal of Psychiatry* 184 (46): 38–44

Hales, D. J., Lozoff, B., Susa, R., Kennell, J.H. (1977) Defining the limits of the maternal sensitive period. *Developmental Medicine and Child Neurology* 19: 454–461

Hammer, R.P., Burton-Jeangros, C. (2013) Tensions around risks in pregnancy: A typology of women's experiences of surveillance medicine. *Social Science & Medicine* 93: 55–63

Hatfield, E. and Rapson, R. (2000) *Rosie*. Pittsburgh, PA: SterlingHouse.

Heerdink, M.W., Van Kleef, G.A., Homan, A.C., Fischer, A.H. (2013) On the social influence of emotions in groups: Interpersonal effects of anger and happiness on conformity versus deviance. *Journal of Personality & Social Psychology* 105 (2): 262–284

House of Commons (1995) *Medical (Professional Performance) Act*. London: HMSO http://www.legislation.gov.uk/ukpga/1995/51/contents accessed 5 May 2014

Kaplan, P.S., Dungan, J.K., Zinser, M.C. (2004) Infants of chronically depressed mothers learn in response to male, but not female, infant directed speech. *Developmental Psychology* 40 (2): 140–148

Kirkham, M. (1999) The culture of midwifery in the National Health Service in England. *Journal of Advanced Nursing* 30 (3): 732–739

Kitzinger, S. (2005) *The Politics of Birth*. Edinburgh: Elsevier

Klaus, M.H., Kennel J.H. (1976) *Maternal-Infant Bonding*. St Louis: C.V. Mosby

Levine, P.A. (2005) *Healing Trauma*. Boulder: Sounds True Inc

MacLellan, J. (2014) Claiming an ethic of care for midwifery. *Nursing Ethics* 21: 1–9 http://nej.sagepub.com/content/early/2014/06/09/0969733014534878.full.pdf+html Accessed 11 August 2014

MacValue, F. (2013) Is midwifery knowledge a relevant construct in contemporary practice? *Essentially MIDIRS* 4 (5): 32–38

Mander, R., Fleming, V. (2002) *Failure to Progress: The contraction of the midwifery profession*. London: Routledge

Menard, J., Brunet, L., Savoie, A. (2011) Interpersonal workplace deviance: Why do offenders act out? A comparative look on personality and organisational variables. *Canadian Journal of Behavioural Science* 43 (4): 309–317

Merton, R.K. (1957) *Social Theory and Social Structure*. Glencoe: Free Press

Merton, R.K., Nisbet, R.A. (eds) (1961) *Contemporary Social Problems*. New York: Harcourt Brace

Meyer, S., Raikes, H.A., Virmani, E.A., Waters, S., Thompson, R.A. (2014) Parent emotion representations and the socialization of emotion regulation in the family. *International Journal of Behavioral Development* 38 (2): 164–173

Nair, V., Chandraharan, E. (2010) Clinical Negligence Scheme for Trusts (CNST) *Obstetrics, Gynaecology & Reproductive Medicine* 20 (4): 125–128

Nishitani, S., Kuwamoto, S., Takahira, A., Miyamura, T., Shinohara, K. (2014) Maternal prefrontal cortex activation by newborn infant odors. *Chemical Senses* http://chemse. oxfordjournals.org/content/early/2014/01/07/chemse.bjt068.full.pdf+html Accessed 3 May 2014

Nissen, E. Uvnas-Moberg, K., Svensson, K., Stock, S., Widstrom, A.M., Winberg, J. (1996) Different patterns of oxytocin, prolactin but not cortisol release during breastfeeding in women delivered by caesarean section or by the vaginal route. *Early Human Development* 45: 103–118

NMC (Nursing and Midwifery Council) (2012) *Midwives Rules and Standards.* London: NMC

NMC (2015) *The Code. Professional Standards of Practice and Behaviour for Nurses and Midwives.* London: NMC. Online: http://www.nmc-uk.org/Documents/NMC-Publications/NMC-Code-A5-FINAL.pdf last accessed February 2015

Odent, M. (1999) *The Scientification of Love.* London: Free Association Books

Odent, M. (2003) *Birth and Breastfeeding.* Clairview Westport: Bergin & Garvey

O'Hara, M.W., McCabe, J.E. (2013) Postpartum depression: Current status and future directions. *Annual Review of Clinical Psychology* 9: 379–407

Olza-Fernandez, I., Gabriel, M.A.M., Gil-Sanchez, A., Garcia-Segura, L.M. (2014) Neuroendocrinology of childbirth and mother-child attachment: The basis of an etiopathogenic model of perinatal neurobiological disorders. *Frontiers in Neuroendocrinology* 36 (3): 279–291

Park, C.S., Yeoum, S.G., Choi, E.S. (2005) Study of subjectivity in the perception of caesarean birth. *Nursing and Health Sciences* 7 (1): 3–8

Parsons, T. (1949) *Essays in Sociological Theory.* New York: Free Press

Parsons, T (1951) *The Social System.* Glencoe: Free Press

Pronin, E., Berger, J., Molouki, S. (2007) Alone in a crowd of sheep: Asymmetric perceptions of conformity and their roots in an introspection illusion. *Journal of Personality and Social Psychology* 92 (4): 585–595

Sox, H.C., Higgins, M.C., Owens, D.K. (2013) *Medical Decision Making.* 2nd edition. Chichester: Wiley-Blackwell

Stewart, M. (2005) 'I'm just going to wash you down': Sanitising the vaginal examination. *Journal of Advanced Nursing* 51 (6): 587–594

Tellis, G.J., Prabhu, J.C., Chandy, R.K. (2009) Radical innovation across nations: The preeminence of corporate culture. *Journal of Marketing* 73 (1): 3–23

Thomas, V., Dixon A. (2012) *Improving Safety in Maternity Services: A toolkit for teams.* London: The Kings Fund

Wadhwa, P.D., Entringer, S., Buss, C., Lu, M.C. (2011) The contribution of maternal stress to preterm birth: Issues and considerations. *Clinics in Perinatology* 38 (3): 351–384

Weber, M. (1947) *The Theory of Social and Economic Organization.* Glencoe: Free Press of Glencoe (Translated by A.M. Henderson and T. Parsons)

Zoghbi-Manrique-de-Lara, P. (2010) Employee deviance as a response to injustice and task-related discontent. *The Psychologist Manager Journal* 13: 131–146

6 Spirituality and midwifery care

Louise Hunter

Aim

This chapter aims to define and explore the concept of spirituality and outline its importance in midwifery care, particularly as a counterbalance to the medical focus on controlling physical (dys)function during childbirth that persists in many maternity care settings. After exposing the shortcomings of the medical approach, it will be argued that spiritual care is at the heart of what midwives do, or would like to be able to do, on a daily basis and has the potential to improve the wellbeing of women and their children, midwives and society as a whole.

Learning outcomes

By the end of this chapter the reader will be able to:

- Articulate the philosophical case against an overly medical approach, particularly in respect to maternity care
- Appreciate the significance of childbirth as a rite of passage with the potential to positively or negatively affect the wellbeing of women, their children and families in the short and longer term
- Appreciate the contribution of the non-rational and unseen to individual and collective wellbeing
- Define spirituality, particularly in terms of interconnectedness and relationships
- Understand the central importance of presence in spiritual care and articulate different ways of being present
- Suggest ways in which midwives might introduce a more spiritual approach into their work, in order to ensure care empowers rather than diminishes women

---

Introduction

Since the publication of the *Changing Childbirth* report (DH, 2003) government documents, together with professional literature from the Nursing and Midwifery Council (NMC) have advocated a holistic, woman- (or patient-) centred approach to care (DH, 2007; NMC, 2015). Increasingly, particularly in nursing literature, such care is seen to incorporate a spiritual dimension (Baldacchino, 2006; Fahy and Hastie, 2008; Hall, 2008; RCN, 2011). Recognition of the need for a more spiritual approach to care and debate about what this should entail led to a call, in 2006, for the establishment of a distinct field of spirituality-in-nursing (Swinton, 2006), and an entire edition of the *Journal of Clinical Nursing* was devoted to the issue. Despite a proliferation of literature on the subject, however, the concept of spirituality remains poorly defined, particularly in relation to midwifery care (Linhares, 2012; Miner-Williams, 200), and nursing and midwifery continue to be dominated by a medical approach that privileges interventions and physical checks (Baker et al., 2005; Swinton, 2006). It is hoped that exploring and defining spirituality and spiritual care, attempting to underpin them with a philosophy and rationale, and outlining their relevance to midwifery practice, will contribute to the formulation of a credible alternative to the culture of scientific reductionism that prevails in many United Kingdom maternity care settings. It might first be in order, however, briefly to outline why such an alternative is necessary.

The rise and rise of technomedicine

The dominant Western medical philosophy was dubbed 'technomedicine' by the American anthropologist Robbie Davis-Floyd (Davis-Floyd, 2001). It is a mind set based on the belief that the body is a machine-like entity inhabited by but entirely separate from the mind. This philosophy dates back to seventeenth-century thinkers such as Descartes, who paved the way for a systematic division of the body into a series of distinct systems that could be investigated, recorded, tested, regulated, controlled and healed through outside manipulation by expert physicians (Davis-Floyd, 1990, 2001: Parratt and Fahy, 2008). There can be no doubt that the medical revolution that Descartes set in motion has resulted in treatments that have been of great benefit to humanity. However, by recognising only what can be measured and seen, and discounting and even demonising alternative outlooks that seek to see and treat people as more than body-machines, medical advances have arguably come at some cost.

The case against technomedicine has been made by philosophers such as Foucault (1989) and Illich (1995). It essentially rests on the premise that technomedicine is not just a means of curing disease but a value system that controls and subjugates both individuals and entire societies (Foucault, 1989). The testing and regulating of body-machines has led to the reduction of a person to an immune system that needs tests and diagnoses to tell it how it should feel (Illich, 1995). Furthermore, progress has come to be measured by the development of ever-more complicated machines to perform more intricate tests and procedures – the process has come to dominate the individuals it is supposed to serve (Davis-Floyd, 2001; Downe and McCourt, 2008).

Application to practice

There are many examples of this trend in midwifery care, and you will probably be able to think of some that you have encountered. Recent instances I have come across include machines for analysing urine dip sticks and portable bilimeters for measuring jaundice levels in the community. While the bilimeters were initially welcomed as potentially circumventing the need for blood tests, the midwives I work with feel that junior colleagues are losing the confidence to assess neonates holistically, and anxious parents are requesting readings on asymptomatic babies, distrusting other signs telling them that their baby is well. Furthermore, the machine can be quite inaccurate, and high readings have to be followed up with a blood test anyway.

As machines proliferate and investigations and interventions increase, the power of technomedicine rises and that of alternative approaches diminishes (Page, 2008). By restricting medical knowledge to white-coated experts, technomedicine has made individuals and societies reliant on its pronouncements and deprived them of the ability to care for and heal themselves (Baker et al., 2005; Illich, 1995). It is therefore in a position of great power, deciding what is normal or desirable, who is sick and what should be done to them (Illich, 1995). Of particular note to midwifery, Illich writes that 'once a society is so organised that people are patients because they are unborn, newborn, menopausal or at some other "age of risk", the population inevitably loses some of its autonomy to its healers' (1995, p. 26). The diminution of the autonomy of both women and midwives caused by the pathologising of normal life events can be seen in the widespread fear and mistrust of home birth in the UK (Essentially MIDIRS, 2014).

The shortcomings of a technomedical approach in maternity care

Far from being 'objective' and 'evidence-based', technomedicine is in fact based on antiquated patriarchal beliefs, evincing a deep mistrust of women's bodies and their life-giving potential. The prototype body-machine is male – female body-machines are inherently deviant, untrustworthy and in need of control (Davis-Floyd, 1990). Furthermore, by basing its entire premise on what can be seen, counted and charted, technomedicine has developed a great fear of what cannot be seen, and does not conform to its efforts to control and regulate (Parratt and Fahy, 2008). It has no answer for the new mother on the postnatal ward, struggling to come to terms with what happened to her during her labour and birth and with how to mother her baby – in fact it does not even recognise her distress, concerning itself instead with her urine output, circulation and mobility level. Moreover, by treating her as a defective machine, technomedicine has in fact sent this mother a series of powerful messages about her position in society and her capabilities – not being regarded as able to give birth on her own, she has been timed and charted. If she failed to contract or dilate at the prescribed rate technomedicine would have stepped in, at all times emphasising the risky process she was undergoing and her need for its expertise. In all probability, it would not have been the woman but technomedicine that decided when she was in labour, and when and whether she was able to give birth unaided. Davis-Floyd drew attention in 1990 to the way in which, at the moment of birth, many women were draped in sterile sheets, graphically illustrating that their babies must be protected from the uncleanliness of the mother's body – this practice still persists in some UK units today. After birth the timing and charting continues, as concerns are expressed about the adequacy of a mother's milk to sustain her infant.

Trigger

Practices such as draping women in sterile sheets are rituals – there is no evidence that they are of any tangible benefit, but they help the practitioner to feel in control and transmit a message about the power and place of both the performer and the recipient. What rituals are you aware of where you practice? What effects do they have on midwives and women?

Within the technomedical paradigm, birth is seen as an event that is safe only in retrospect, and that is judged solely on the physical wellbeing of mother and baby (Baker et al., 2005). Technomedicine assumes that, given a particular treatment, every body-machine will react in a similar way – hence its development of the randomised controlled trial, which seeks to prove the effectiveness of an intervention by minimising surrounding 'noise'. However, not only does it increasingly appear the case that bodies, just like other scientific matter, react in different ways in different environments (see Downe and McCourt, 2008 for an in-depth discussion of this phenomenon), but people are more than body-machines – they are, as other chapters in this book show, sociological (Chapter 1), psychological (Chapter 3) and political beings (Chapter 8) who interact with each other and with their surroundings. Birth is not only a biological process but a social, emotional and spiritual event, the outcome of which depends on a host of interacting physiological, cultural, environmental and psychological factors (Downe and McCourt, 2008; Lewis and McCaffery, 2000). Trying to reduce it to a predictable biological phenomenon potentially endangers the physical as well as the emotional, spiritual and psychological wellbeing of mother and baby (Downe and McCourt, 2008; Parratt and Fahy, 2008; Swinton, 2006). The effects of this approach are seen in the widespread anxiety and stress experienced by many new mothers (Baker et al., 2005; McCourt 2006). Suicide is now a leading cause of maternal death in the first six months after birth (CMACE, 2011). Moreover, the physical safety that technomedical care promises labouring women is an illusion – for example, once it passes a certain point, the caesarean section rate ceases to improve, and may even have a negative impact on, maternal and neonatal morbidity and mortality rates (Wagner, 2001). The World Health Organization (WHO) therefore recommends that caesarean section rates should not exceed 15 per cent (WHO, 2009).

Ignoring the wider significance of childbirth affects not only individuals but entire communities: if people are treated as dependent machines they are more likely to act as such, and not develop the resources necessary to nurture life in themselves and others (Downe and McCourt, 2008; Redshaw, 2006). The way a woman is treated during and after childbirth will shape and influence her experiences as a mother, affecting not only her physical health but also her sense of self and competence (McCourt, 2006: Page, 2008; Pembroke and Pembroke, 2008). Odent (1999) in particular has argued that the hormonal responses that are induced in both mother and baby at this time will affect their capacity to love and therefore the way they interact with each other and go on to interact with society at large (see also Chapter 5 of this book).

Spirituality: An alternative approach

Care around the time of birth affects, then, not only the physical but also the metaphysical wellbeing of individuals and communities. Although it includes psychological, sociological and cultural elements, this metaphysical wellbeing is perhaps more completely encapsulated in the concept of spirituality. Davis-Floyd (2008, p. xi) writes that 'spirit does exist ... and to ignore it in the healing process is to leave out the most important element in illness and facilitator of wellness'. Although spirituality is widely held to have an impact on health and wellbeing, it is somewhat taboo, perhaps because it cannot be contained in the language of scientific orthodoxy, and health practitioners, including midwives, are unsure how to incorporate it into their practice (Hall, 2013; Swinton, 2006). Midwifery literature on spirituality tends to become somewhat flowery and poetical, leaving it open to ridicule from the orthodoxy it is seeking to challenge. What follows below is therefore an attempt to define spirituality, and outline the principles of spiritual care, in a language that is acceptable and makes sense to a culture steeped in the values of rational scientific thought.

Spirituality as 'inner life'

While technomedicine concerns itself with outward, tangible signs of wellbeing, spirituality explores the intangible, inner life. It equates to the non-rational (as opposed to 'irrational') ways of being and knowing identified by Parratt and Fahy (2008). The notion of an inner, spiritual self is fundamental to much Eastern philosophy (Chan et al., 2006), and resonates strongly with the conscious and unconscious minds proposed by psychoanalysts such as Carl Jung (Jung, 1968). Spiritualists contend that the inner self or spirit encapsulates the essence of being human and provides meaning to life (Callister and Khalaf, 2010; Chan et al., 2006; Hall, 2013; Miner-Williams, 2006). Insofar as it represents the essence of an individual, spirit is sometimes referred to as a person's soul (Hall, 2006). To ignore or suppress it is to be at best incomplete and at worst demeaned and broken. Realising our full potential (some would even say 'being fully alive') necessitates balancing and connecting the physical and spiritual sides of our existence (Chan et al., 2006).

Spirituality as relatedness

Spirituality is about more than the inner life of individuals, however. It also contends that people do not exist in isolation but through relatedness with others and with their environments (Hall, 2008; Swinton 2006). Spiritual wellbeing is enhanced and even instigated through validating relationships with other people or with the natural world. Reed (1992) describes how relatedness can be experienced intrapersonally (as a connectedness within the self), interpersonally (with others or nature) and transpersonally (with a power outside and greater than the self). Hall (2008) also points out that such relatedness can cross time, as a connection with past or future experiences, events or people. Spirituality involves being connected and connecting to something that is at one and the same time located within and outside the self – Pembroke and Pembroke (2008) describe it as having both an immanent and a transcendent form.

The idea that humans are only truly whole when they are connected to an essential otherness in the universe, and that relationships with other people or with the natural world somehow give access to or even create this otherness, is at the heart of much Eastern and Western religious thought. Indeed, its resonance with religion is perhaps what makes many health professionals, who are trained and educated to follow the precepts of rationality and science, so uncomfortable about acknowledging and discussing spirituality. It has been suggested that religious spirituality should be separated from secular spirituality, as trying to relate the two results in vague, 'one size fits all' precepts and definitions that are ultimately meaningless (Hall, 2008; Swinton, 2006). However, although the expression of spirituality might vary between individuals and cultures, the underlying ideas are remarkably similar (Miner-Williams, 2006), and there is surely much to be learned from, and much illuminating discussion to be had between, people from different religious and secular traditions. Indeed, as Downe and McCourt (2008) have shown, ideas of interconnectivity owe as much to cutting-edge science as to ancient religion. This resonance surely adds to, rather than detracts from, their credibility.

Spirituality as a connecting and collective energy

What then is this inside/outside, essence/otherness, that is so essential to human wellbeing? Fahy and Hastie (2008, p. 26) describe it as that 'energetic, electromagnetic part of self which existed prior to conception and which is part of universal energy'. The belief, implicit in this statement, that communion with spiritual 'otherness' is personally energising and enriching because we are connecting to the whole from which we were formed goes back at least to Saint Augustine (354–430) in Christian thought (Augustine of Hippo, 1984). Spiritual energy is 'integrative' (Miner-Williams, 2006), connecting that which already is, and creative – a 'life force'. In Western theology, the spirit is the 'breath of life' (Hall, 2006). It is also associated with wisdom, and humility in the recognition that, as an individual, one is a small part of a much greater whole (Jung, 1968). Despite its energetic and life-giving potential, spirituality and spiritual experiences are often associated with stillness and calm. Spiritual presence or energy is felt in quiet, contemplative moments, often at the end of a quest or in and around pivotal, life-changing events (Jung, 1968; Miner-Williams, 2006).

In Western scientific and secular thinking, such was the stranglehold of Descartes' ideas that it was not until the advent of psychoanalysis in the early twentieth century that the role of the spirit in wellbeing was established. Jung, one of the founders of psychoanalysis, proposed that the mind was made up of conscious and unconscious thoughts, both of which could influence physical wellbeing. The unconscious mind consists of a personal unconscious (the thoughts and actions an individual has forgotten or deliberately repressed) and a collective unconscious in which everyone shares and that has existed since the genesis of the human race (Jung, 1968). Jung cited the almost universal parallelism of mythological motifs as proof of the collective unconsciousness' existence. He argued that it crosses space and time and belongs to all people, although they experience it in culturally conditioned ways (Jung, 1968). The collective unconscious is inherited in the shape of thought structures and 'possibilities of thoughts', and is encountered in dreams and symbols that Jung noted feature strongly at crucial transitional periods of life such as birth, death or initiation into a new stage of existence. For Jung the dreams and symbols encountered by people at these transformative moments represented attempts by their unconscious minds to make accessible the ways and patterns with which humanity has historically coped with such transitions. To ignore them was to risk an incomplete initiation, and to become alienated from the personal as well as the collective self.

Spirituality: A feminine quality?

It is also possible to argue that spirituality is a uniquely feminine concept. In fact, Hall (2008) goes so far as to suggest that women may be more spiritual than men, in that the beliefs and behaviours that tend to result from a connection to others and to one's environment, such as compassion and non-violence, are more often associated with women. Men such as Nelson Mandela and Mahatma Gandhi perhaps challenge this view, however. From a Jungian perspective, both men and women are a mix of different traits, some of which are traditionally viewed as masculine and others as feminine. In Western society, traits viewed as feminine, such as vague feelings and moods, prophetic hunches and receptiveness to the irrational (or non-rational) have been viewed as inferior, along with women themselves, while more acceptable, rational personality traits have been seen as male (also see Chapter 4). Jung argues that the privileging of the rational, conscious, 'male' side of humanity at the expense of the non-rational and unconscious has led to the creation of a society where individuals feel alienated from their true selves, from each other and from their environment.

To be whole, in Eastern and in Jungian thought, is to balance the physical and spiritual, rational and non-rational, sides of existence. This balance is increasingly associated with health and wellbeing, and an ability to integrate and cope with life events (Baldacchino, 2006; Chan et al 2006). Spiritual wellbeing through meditation is a central component of Mindfulness (Chan et al., 2006), which is becoming a popular and widely used therapy in health and social care.

Birth as a time of spiritual growth

Giving birth and becoming a mother is widely held to involve a transition from one state of being to another, with potential for personal development and spiritual growth (Hall, 2013; Parratt, 2008). Transitions are traditionally associated with danger as well as enrichment, as in order to become something other an individual must leave the safety of the known and cross a liminal no-mans' land before being incorporated back into society as a different self (McCourt, 2006; Parratt, 2008). The liminal period, when a person is neither their old self nor quite their new one, is a time of great vulnerability during which, unprotected by a fully formed identity, people are exposed and impressionable.

Application to practice

The early postnatal period is a liminal time in which many new mothers feel unconfident, sensitive and vulnerable. For example, young mothers in my recent study of feeding experiences described being particularly sensitive to things that were said or done to them on the postnatal ward (Hunter, 2014):

'I felt maybe [the midwife] was talking down to me . . . and 'cos I was quite emotional anyway, it just made me like – quite teary and stuff . . . [but] most probably it wasn't her, it was most probably just – just the way I was at the time.'

Across cultures, humans have sought to control, contain and manage the passage of transition through ritual or spiritual practices (McCourt, 2006). These rites of passage are designed safely to convey an individual from one social state to another, and to impress on them society's expectations of their new role (Davis-Floyd, 1990). Parratt writes that spiritual practices 'guide people toward connectivity and integration despite the disconnections of change' (2008, p30). However, as discussed earlier, Davis-Floyd has shown that modern obstetric practice is peppered with rituals that disempower and subjugate birthing women by emphasising their dependence on technomedical expertise. Such practices transmit powerful messages about the power and place of women as mothers and are held by some to impact negatively on their wellbeing (Parratt, 2008). Parratt and Walsh argue that midwives need to replace such rituals with the 'ordinary practices of life' (Parratt, 2008, p. 40) that connect us to our environment and to each other – such as simply being there, sharing stories, or making tea (Parratt, 2008; Walsh, 2007).

Application to practice

The young women in my research on feeding experiences particularly appreciated midwives who spent time with them, and spoke of how this helped them gain confidence in their abilities. The following exchange illustrates the importance of chatting:

Avril: I remember, when I was there [in hospital], there used to be a midwife – she used to come in about half eight, nine every night, and she used to just close the little – you know the little window thing – she used to close that and come and sit down . . . and talk to me – it'd be about everything sort of thing . . .

Children's Centre Worker: And all those little things just become so important don't they?

Avril: A little talk, 'cos it does help like.

Children's Centre Worker: . . . I think we lose that sometimes, don't we, in our busyness.

Midwifery and spirituality

In her enduringly popular book, *Spiritual Midwifery*, Ina May Gaskin describes birth as a 'sacrament' (1990, p. 1), underlining its significance as a metaphysical transition as well as a physical event. Midwifery has long been held to be about more than just physical care. In France, a midwife is a *sage-femme* – a wise woman (a spiritual trait), and in Anglo Saxon she is of course 'with woman'. Relationships and relatedness are held to lie at the heart of midwifery practice, as well as being at the core of spirituality (Curtis et al., 2006: McCourt, 2006: Page, 2008). The capacity of midwives to be with and guide women through birth has historically been demonised as witchcraft – secret, non-rational, spiritual knowledge and ritual powers that threatened the ordered, rational world (Lahood, 2007). More recently, many midwives working in the National Health Service (NHS) have been prevented from carrying out supposedly deviant practices, such as being with and relating to women, by a rigid medical hierarchy and an overstretched service that prioritises routine observations and checks. Indeed Page (2008) has argued that technomedicine has such a stranglehold over much maternity care that midwives need to learn to work 'with woman' again, rather than 'with institution'.

Spiritual midwifery care: Empowering presence

Spiritual midwifery care seeks to redress the imbalance caused by technomedicine by recognising and addressing the metaphysical aspects of birth as a rite of passage. It acknowledges that, in addition to meeting a woman's physical needs, the midwife's role involves helping mothers to grow into and embrace their new identities, and connect to the world and people around them in their new roles. Spiritual care seeks to address women's physical, emotional, social and spiritual needs through relationships centred on the concepts of presence and empowerment.

The concept of presence is central to spiritual care. Presence is defined as a way of being there or standing with another, especially during a challenging time (Melnechenko,

2003; Zyblock, 2010). It involves being available to respond to a person's needs, and 'the sharing of oneself through full attention to the other' (Melnechenko, 2003, p. 19). Midwives who are present are able to connect with women in a way that creates a safe, reassuring, calm space that helps them cope with the challenges they are facing (whether these be during pregnancy, birth or adapting postnatally) (Pembroke and Pembroke, 2008; Zyblock, 2010). A midwife who is truly present is able to hold a situation and an individual in such a way that the former feels manageable and the latter capable. Presence enables people to find a way through a challenging situation (Zyblock, 2010).

Application to practice

I was introduced to the concept of holding by a woman I looked after ante and postnatally through two pregnancies. At the beginning of her second pregnancy, she opted for a home birth because, despite giving birth to her first child in an alongside midwifery-led unit, where everyone had been very kind, she 'just didn't feel very held by the midwives'. This comment really made me reflect on the ways that I had been present with labouring women.

The concept of presence has been explored in the context of nursing care. Osterman et al. (2010) describe four different types of nursing presence:

- Absent presence: the nurse is physically present, but totally self-absorbed and not interacting or connecting with the patient.
- Partial presence: the nurse is physically present, but focusing on tasks and not on the patient themselves. This has been found to be the default mode of some midwives on busy postnatal wards (Hunter, 2014).
- Full presence: the nurse is physically and psychologically present, interacting with and focusing on the patient. S/he is caring and empathetic.
- Transcendent or spiritual presence: the focus is on being there, rather than completing tasks (Baldacchino, 2006). The nurse is grounded, focused on, and holding, the patient. The connection between the nurse and patient creates an almost palpable energy field (Davis-Floyd, 2001), and the nurse's presence is felt by the patient as peaceful and comforting.

Full and spiritual presence are perhaps on a continuum – full presence becomes spiritual presence when such presence is needed and when the participants and environment allow this to happen.

Spiritual midwifery care and different ways of knowing

Towards the spiritual end of the continuum, both full and spiritual presence also open up the possibility of different ways of knowing. Osterman et al. (2010) acknowledge that when a nurse is fully present, in a calm and quiet space, with a patient they are better able critically to assess their needs. By being fully or spiritually present nurses and midwives are able to assess and respond to a situation in ways that are not possible if only the rational, task checking, part of the mind is being used. Full or spiritual presence utilises unconscious, intuitive, instinctive and non-rational, as well as conscious and rational, knowing. Intuitive and instinctive knowing have long been dismissed by the rational, scientific community. Indeed, evidence-based practice is often held to have been introduced to replace such primitive and unreliable ways of practising (Rees, 2011). However, there is also an argument that intuition is a mark of the expert practitioner, reacting to subtle changes or cues and subconsciously processing a wealth of knowledge, experience and understanding in order to determine how to act (Benner, 1984). The renowned scientist James Lovelock points out that intuition has been crucial in scientific breakthroughs, and argues that, as both intuition and reason are part of our evolutionary past, both are necessary for our future survival. He uses the example of catching a ball to illustrate that intuitive thought is, in fact, far quicker than rational thought. Although we are trained to catch balls, and can practice this skill, the act of catching is never done rationally or consciously, as our conscious brains are far too slow (Lovelock, 2014). If we consciously told our limbs to move in this or that direction, the ball would either have hit us or sailed past before we'd raised an arm. Furthermore, scientific fields such as quantum physics, and advances in our understanding of areas such as physiology, have shown that rational cause and effect thinking only gets us so far – it simply cannot explain everything. Life is infinitely more complicated than previously thought, and involves the continuous interaction of vast arrays of non-linear systems (Lovelock, 2014). In order to grasp the whole it is increasingly necessary to use unconscious, non-rational, knowing. According to Lovelock, 'humanity badly needs to know that an inability to explain something rationally does not deny its existence' (2014, p. 79). It would appear that the art of being present and knowing might have uses beyond patient care.

> **Trigger**
>
> Reflect on an encounter you have had in practice. What different ways of knowing did you use to inform the way you acted and the decisions you made? If you are a student, ask your mentor what informed his or her actions in a given situation.

Spiritual midwifery care and empowerment

Importantly, being spiritually present does not require one to have all the answers, but to give a woman or patient the space and courage to find their own way (Miner-Williams, 2006). At its core in midwifery is the fundamental and unshakable conviction that women can almost always give birth themselves, and that they each carry within them the potential to become confident and capable mothers. Spiritual midwives are not afraid of birth, they believe in the process and in their own ability to respond appropriately to unfolding events.

| Trigger |

If you are a student, try and work with an independent midwife or a mentor who works in more spiritual ways. Such people usually have an incredibly in-depth knowledge of physiology and the evidence that informs their practice. This gives them a level of confidence and expertise that is perhaps missing among practitioners who rely on guidelines and protocols to tell them what to do.

Illich (1995) observes that, when cities are built around vehicles, they devalue human feet. Thus while technomedicine, however inadvertently, emphasises human (and particularly female) incapacity and dependence, spiritual care has the potential to transform and liberate. Women who are enabled to find and use their own power as they become mothers may then be able to use that power in other areas of their lives (Parratt, 2008). Davis-Floyd quotes a mother who was able to be in control of her own birthing experience at home as saying 'I realised that if I could do that great thing, perhaps I could do other things as well' (1990, p. 183). This contrasts strongly with the following statement from a woman in a study by Behruzi et al. (2011, p.11) who gave birth in a highly medicalised hospital: 'I would not be able to deal with a normal delivery, I am not capable'.

By being with, believing in and empowering women, spiritual midwifery care is centred on the concept of salutogenesis – the creation of wellness (Davis-Floyd, 2008). It is thus a more holistic approach than technomedicine, which focuses on correcting illness and deviance. Again this concept aligns with Eastern healing traditions, which aim to resolve problems by focusing on strength and synergy rather than homing in on weakness and cutting out individual symptoms (Chan et al., 2006). Central to the concept of salutogenesis is coherence. A salutogenic approach recognises that physiology and wellbeing are influenced by a web of cultural, social, environmental and psychological factors (Downe and McCourt, 2008). Coherence, which builds resilience to adverse events, results when all these factors are working together (Downe, 2010). Thus midwives are able positively to influence physiology and wellbeing by being present with a woman, providing a safe environment and enabling her to feel stronger emotionally.

Challenges to providing spiritual midwifery care

It would be a tall order for midwives to be spiritually present all the time. In their research with oncology nurses, Osterman et al. (2010) report that the nurses were present in different ways within single interactions. Spiritual care, however, is open to the possibility of spiritual presence, and able to use it to provide emotional support. The nursing literature suggests that such presence provides comfort, motivation, hope and enhanced healing (Zyblock, 2010).

The concepts of salutogenesis, connectedness and the Jungian 'collective self', which are all contained within spirituality and spiritual care, indicate that it is about more than isolated encounters between individuals and carers. It is also about the environment in which care is given and, some would argue, the society that sanctions that care. It is extremely difficult for individual midwives to be fully, let alone spiritually, present with women in busy, overstretched units where medical tasks are given priority and midwives are stressed, undervalued and preoccupied with their own problems. Furthermore, it is virtually impossible to promote groundedness and coherence in others if one lacks those qualities oneself (Baldacchino, 2006; Pemboroke and Pembroke, 2008). It is argued that an overly technomedical service has a negative impact on midwives as well as women (Page, 2008), and that the pressure to become a cog in the technomedical wheel is a reason that many midwives leave the profession (Curtis et al., 2006).

Trigger

What might be the barriers to providing spiritual care where you work? How might they be overcome?

If midwives recognise the importance of spiritual care, and their role in providing such care, then they need to create a working environment that fosters and encourages a belief in the birthing process and in women's capabilities. There is evidence that this has been happening in the UK in recent years in the proliferation of alongside birthing units (Walsh, 2007). However, a recent observational study conducted on a postnatal ward suggested that midwives lack control of their time and space within more medical environments, and there is much work to be done before spiritual care becomes the norm here (Hunter, 2014).

The importance of balance

It has been argued in this chapter that spirituality is everything that technomedicine is not. Where technomedicine studies and observes, spirituality relates. Technomedicine cures, spirituality enables. Technomedicine is powerful and clever, spirituality is humble and wise. Technomedics do, spiritualists are. However, it has also been pointed out that wholeness (or coherence) is about balancing the physical and spiritual, rational and non-rational sides of the self (Jung, 1968; Parratt, 2008). This balance also applies to communities and to society. Downe (2010) writes that it has become almost taken for granted within midwifery that medical is 'bad' and midwifery is 'good'. She argues for a need to unite the two, pointing out that places with low rates of caesarean sections and good morbidity and mortality figures tend to have teams that work well together. Davis-Floyd has argued that combining technocratic, humanistic (relational) and holistic (in which she includes spiritual) paradigms would create an opportunity to develop 'the most effective obstetrical system ever known' (2001, p. S5). However, for any kind of balance to be achieved, midwives need to claim and assert their power as the guardians of normal birth and adaptation to parenthood (Fahy and Hastie, 2008; Hunter, 2014). Both obstetricians and midwives also need to recognise and value the abilities of women to determine their own way.

Conclusion

In outlining the two paradigms of technomedical and spiritual care this chapter begs the question, put by Davis-Floyd some time ago, 'who do we want to make ourselves become through the kinds of healthcare we create?' (2001, p. 21). It has been argued that technomedical maternity care ignores the significance of birth as a time of transformation and undermines women's strength and capabilities. Spiritual care, by contrast, allows for the possibility of enabling women to realise their own power and potential as creators and healers. It promotes connection with the unconscious, the non-rational, the life force – alienation from which, according to Jung, is at root of Western society's alienation from itself (Jung, 1968). Attending to the spiritual as well as the physical events around childbearing restores a balance that promotes wellness and can help people to heal themselves (Chan et al., 2006). Spiritual care is a holistic approach that uses intuitive and instinctive, as well as rational, ways of knowing and seeks to relate to, connect with and empower women through presence. In order to embed spiritual care in midwifery practice, midwives need to create a working environment that facilitates relationships, that believes in and fosters the capabilities of women, and trusts its own ability to act appropriately in the event of a problem. Spiritual care is about personal strength and groundedness and, to paraphrase Gaskin, the ability not to be afraid. Such an approach is likely to reach beyond the childbearing period to affect the way mothers adapt, cope and relate to their families and the wider community.

References

Augustine of Hippo (1984). *City of God.* St Ives: Penguin.

Baker S, Choi P, Henshaw C and Tree J (2005). '"I felt as though I'd been in jail": women's experiences of maternity care during labour, delivery and the immediate postpartum'. *Feminism and Psychology* 15:3, 315–42.

Baldacchino D (2006). 'Nursing competencies for spiritual care'. *Journal of Clinical Nursing* 15:7, 885–96.

Behruzi R, Hatem M, Goulet L and Fraser W (2011). 'The facilitating factors and barriers encountered in the adoption of a humanized birth care approach in a highly specialized university affiliated hospital'. *BMC Women's Health* 11: 53.

Benner P (1984). *From Novice to Expert: Excellence and power in clinical nursing practice.* California: Addison-Wesley.

Callister L and Khalaf I (2010). 'Spirituality in childbearing women'. *The Journal of Perinatal Education* 19:2, 16–24.

CMACE (Centre for Maternal and Child Enquiries) (2011). 'Saving Mothers' Lives: Reviewing maternal deaths to make motherhood safer: 2006–2008. The Eighth Report of the Confidential Enquiries into Maternal Deaths in the United Kingdom'. *British Journal of Obstetrics and Gynaecology* 118, Supplement 1, 1–203.

Chan C, Ng S, Ho R and Chow A (2006). 'East meets West: Applying spirituality in clinical practice'. *Journal of Clinical Nursing* 15:7, 822–32.

Curtis P, Ball L and Kirkham M (2006). 'Why do midwives leave? (Not) being the kind of midwife you want to be'. *British Journal of Midwifery* 14:1, 27–31.

Davis-Floyd R (1990). 'The role of obstetrical rituals'. *Social Science and Medicine* 31:2, 175–89.

Davis-Floyd R (2001). 'The technocratic, humanistic and holistic paradigms of childbirth'. *International Journal of Gynecology and Obstetrics* 75, S5–23.

Davis-Floyd R (2008). 'Foreword'. In Downe S (Ed.) *Normal Childbirth: Evidence and debate*. Second edition. Edinburgh: Churchill Livingstone, p. ix–xv.

DH (Department of Health) (2003). *Changing Childbirth Part 1: Report of the Expert Maternity Group*. London: DH.

DH (2007). *Maternity Matters: Choice, access and continuity of care in a safe service*. London: DH.

Downe S and McCourt C (2008). 'From being to becoming: Reconstructing childbirth knowledges'. In Downe S (Ed.) *Normal Childbirth: Evidence and debate*. Second edition. Edinburgh: Churchill Livingstone, p. 3–27.

Downe S (2010). 'Towards salutogenic birth in the twenty first century'. In Downe S and Walsh D (Eds) *Essential Midwifery Practice*. Oxford: Wiley Blackwell, p 289–95.

Essentially MIDIRS (2014). 'Muddying the water'. *Essentially MIDIRS* 5:6, 13.

Fahy K and Hastie C (2008). 'Midwifery guardianship: Reclaiming the sacred in birth'. In Fahy K, Foureur M and Hastie C (Eds) *Birth Territory and Midwifery Guardianship. Theory for practice, education and research*. Edinburgh: Churchill Livingstone, p 21–37.

Foucault M (1989). *The Birth of the Clinic*. Abingdon: Routledge.

Gaskin I (1990). *Spiritual Midwifery*. Third edition. Summertown: The Book Publishing Company.

Hall J (2006). 'Spirituality at the beginning of life'. *Journal of Clinical Nursing* 15:7, 804–10.

Hall J (2008). 'Birth and Spirituality'. In Downe S (Ed.) *Normal Childbirth: Evidence and debate*. Second edition. Edinburgh: Churchill Livingstone, p. 47–63.

Hall J (2010). 'Spirituality and labour care'. In Downe S and Walsh D (Eds): *Essential Midwifery Practice*. Oxford: Wiley Blackwell, p. 235–51.

Hall J (2013). 'Spiritual care: Enhancing meaning in pregnancy and birth'. *The Practising Midwife*, December, 26–27.

Hunter L (2014). Supporting teenage mothers to initiate breastfeeding and developing a support intervention to increase breastfeeding rates in a vulnerable group – the importance of place. Unpublished PhD thesis. London: University of West London.

Illich I (1995). *Limits to Medicine. Medical nemesis: the expropriation of health*. London: Marion Boyars.

Jung C (1968). *The Archetypes and the Collective Unconscious*. Second edition. London: Routledge and Kegan Paul.

Lahood G (2007). 'Rumour of angels and heavenly midwives: Anthropology of transpersonal events and childbirth'. *Women and Birth* 20, 3–10.

Lewis G and McCaffery P (2000). 'Sociological factors affecting the medicalization of midwifery'. In Van Teijlingen E, Lewis G, McCaffery P and Porter M (Eds) *Midwifery and the Medicalization of Childbirth: Comparative perspectives*. New York: Nova.

Linhares C (2012). 'The lived experience of midwives with spirituality in childbirth: Mana from heaven'. *Journal of Midwifery and Women's Health* 57, 165–71.

Lovelock J (2014). *A Rough Ride to the Future*. London: Penguin Books.

McCourt C (2006). 'Becoming a parent'. In Page L and McCandlish R (Eds) *The New Midwifery: Science and sensitivity in practice*. Second edition. Edinburgh: Churchill Livingstone, p. 49–71.

Melnechenko K (2003). 'To make a difference: Nursing presence'. *Nursing Forum* 38:2, 18–24.

Miner-Williams D (2006). 'Putting a puzzle together: Making spirituality meaningful for nursing using an evolving theoretical framework'. *Journal of Clinical Nursing* 15, 811–21.

NMC (Nursing and Midwifery Council) (2015). *The Code. Professional Standards of Practice and Behaviour for Nurses and Midwives*. London: NMC. Online: http://www.nmc-uk.org/Documents/NMC-Publications/NMC-Code-A5-FINAL.pdf last accessed February 2015

Odent M (1999). *The Scientification of Love*. London: Free Association Books.

Osterman P, Scwartz-Barcott D and Asselin M (2010). 'An exploratory study of nurses' presence in daily care on an oncology unit'. *Nursing Forum* 45:3, 197–205.

Page L (2008). 'Being a midwife to midwifery: transforming midwifery services'. In Fahy K, Foureur M and Hastie C (Eds) *Birth Territory and Midwifery Guardianship. Theory for practice, education and research*. Edinburgh: Churchill Livingstone, p. 115–29.

Parratt J (2008). 'Territories of the self and spiritual practices during childbirth'. In Fahy K, Foureur M and Hastie C (Eds) *Birth Territory and Midwifery Guardianship. Theory for practice, education and research*. Edinburgh: Churchill Livingstone, p. 39–54.

Parratt J and Fahy K (2008). 'Including the nonrational is sensible midwifery'. *Women and Birth* 21, 37–42.

Pembroke N and Pembroke J (2008). 'The spirituality of presence in midwifery care'. *Midwifery* 24, 321–27.

RCN (Royal College of Nursing) (2011). *Spirituality in Nursing Care: A pocket guide*. London: RCN.

Redshaw M (2006). 'First relationships and the growth of love and commitment'. In Page L and McCandlish R (Eds) *The New Midwifery: Science and sensitivity in practice*. Second edition. Edinburgh: Churchill Livingstone, p 21–47.

Reed P (1992). 'An emerging paradigm for the investigation of spirituality in nursing'. *Research in Nursing and Health* 15, 349–57.

Rees C (2011). *An Introduction to Research for Midwives*. Edinburgh: Churchill Livingstone.

Swinton J (2006). 'Identity and resistance: Why spiritual care needs "enemies"'. *Journal of Clinical Nursing* 15, 918–28.

Swinton J and McSherry W (2006). 'Editorial'. *Journal of Clinical Nursing* 15, 801–02.

Wagner M (2001). 'Fish can't see the water: The need to humanize birth'. *International Journal of Gynecology and Obstetrics* 75, S25–37.

Walsh D (2007). 'A birth centre's encounters with discourses of childbirth: How resistance led to innovation'. *Sociology of Health and Illness* 29:2, 216–32.

WHO (World Health Organzation) (2009). *Monitoring Emergency Obstetric Care: A handbook*. Geneva: WHO.

Zyblock D (2010). 'Nursing presence in contemporary nursing practice'. *Nursing Forum* 45:2, 120–24.

<table>
<tr><td>7</td></tr>
</table>

Consent, choice and childbirth

Elizabeth Prochaska

Aim

The aim of this chapter is to explain the role of the principle of consent in maternity care, including its philosophical and moral basis in human autonomy and its protection in the English legal system. The chapter reveals how the principle of consent gives rise to a positive obligation on caregivers to provide evidence-based care and to offer women genuine choice about their treatment. It suggests that the principle of informed consent only operates successfully in the context of a respectful relationship between the woman and caregiver that is based on broader principles of human dignity and respectful care. It illustrates the principles with case studies on common aspects of maternity care.

Learning outcomes

By the end of this chapter the reader will be able to:

- Understand the moral and ethical basis for the principle of consent
- Explain how consent is protected by the English legal system
- Appreciate the relationship between consent and choice
- Understand how lack of mental capacity affects consent
- Understand the right to evidence-based care
- Explain how the principles apply in practice

Introduction

Consent is the moral and legal bedrock on which all medical practice rests. Without a person's consent, a professional caregiver does not have legal authority to perform examinations or provide treatment. The principle of consent puts the patient at the centre of decisions about their care and a caregiver cannot be held legally responsible for failing to provide care if the patient has taken an informed decision to decline it. The principle is easily stated, but widely overlooked in maternity care in which woman are frequently subject to 'routine' procedures– such as antenatal screening, vaginal examinations, amniotomy and electronic fetal monitoring – based on hospital policies that sideline the need for individuals to give their consent. Research has shown that a significant proportion of women believe that their consent for medical interventions was not obtained during childbirth. The impact on women of failure to obtain consent for invasive procedures at a time of great vulnerability can be profound and lead to psychological trauma. This chapter introduces the philosophical rationale behind the principle of consent, its manifestation in the legal system and suggests a more sophisticated way of conceptualising consent as a positive right to evidence-based care and choice in healthcare. Ultimately, consent cannot stand apart from broader principles of respectful care. Relationships between mothers and caregivers must be guided by principles of dignity, respect, trust and compassion to ensure that women's decisions are properly supported and care providers do not face criticism for unwanted care.

What is the rationale for the principle of consent?

The principle of human autonomy offers the basic premise for requiring that a person gives their consent to any medical investigation or treatment. An autonomous person is one who is able to make her own decisions free from coercion. Autonomy recognises that each person may make different decisions faced with similar facts; it is an expression of individualism. So long as we accept that autonomy is a fundamental human characteristic that is worthy of protection, it is necessary to give the principle of consent pre-eminence in medical doctrine and practice.

In the context of pregnancy, autonomy might appear to lose some of its potency. It is not necessary to be 'pro-life' to believe that the fetus has value as a potential human life and that pregnant women bear a burden of responsibility for protecting the fetus that they carry. However, pregnancy does not alter a woman's status as equally deserving of respect as a human being. It does not make women less capable of making decisions for themselves. Moral (or medical) disquiet at the choices that a woman makes cannot justify legal sanctions that would imperil her autonomy. In this way, a pregnant woman is no different from a person who makes a healthcare decision that does not benefit another person, such as a father deciding not to donate a kidney to his sick child. His decision might be morally questionable, but he would not be compelled to sacrifice his own bodily integrity for the sake of another.

In practice, different societies give different weight to women's autonomy in pregnancy, depending on their perspective on the value of fetal life. In the Republic of Ireland, for example, the Eighth Amendment to the Irish Constitution protects the right to life of the unborn 'with due regard to the equal right to life of the mother' and women can be lawfully forced to accept medical interventions said to be needed to protect the life of their fetus. But most countries do not, at least officially, dilute the principle of consent in pregnancy. In the United Kingdom, the principles of autonomy and consent are absolute: women who have mental capacity are entitled to make their own decisions about medical care in pregnancy and childbirth.

Trigger

Look up the case of *S v St George's Healthcare Trust* and consider how the legal system protects women's physical autonomy.

How does the English legal system protect the principle of consent?

The English legal system protects the principle of consent in a number of ways. In the common law (the part of English law that is derived from judicial precedent), non-consented medical treatment constitutes the crime of battery and the tort of trespass to the person. An individual who has been subject to medical interference against their will can bring a civil action for damages. A caregiver could also be deemed negligent if they failed to obtain a person's consent to treatment.

The same principles apply to the forcible treatment of pregnant women. In *S v St George's Healthcare Trust*, the Court of Appeal considered the case of a woman detained under the Mental Health Act 1983 who was suffering from pre-eclampsia and had refused a caesarean section. She had been assessed by a psychiatrist and deemed to have mental capacity to make decisions for herself. The hospital applied to the High Court for an urgent order authorising the doctors to perform a caesarean without the woman's consent. The court was told, wrongly, that the woman was in labour and the order was required as a matter of 'life and death'. The Court granted the order without hearing any legal representations on the woman's behalf. After the operation was performed, the woman appealed to the Court of Appeal. The Court's decision forcefully asserted the right of pregnant women to decide for themselves whether to undergo medical treatment:

> . . . while pregnancy increases the personal responsibilities of a woman, it does not diminish her entitlement to decide whether or not to undergo medical treatment. Although human, and protected by the law in a number of different ways . . . an unborn child is not a separate person from its mother. Its need for medical assistance does not prevail over her rights. She is entitled not to be forced to submit to an invasion of her body against her will, whether her own life or that of her unborn child depends on it. Her right is not reduced or diminished merely because her decision to exercise it may appear morally repugnant.

The case resolved any question about the necessity for consent for medical treatment from pregnant women in English law. Women with mental capacity cannot be compelled to accept any form of medical care or treatment during pregnancy and birth.

Consent and mental capacity

A series of recent cases in England has revealed the limits of the principle of consent for pregnant women with mental health disorders who lack mental capacity to give their consent to treatment. Mental capacity is assessed by reference to the test in the Mental Capacity Act 2005, which states that a person lacks capacity when an impairment of, or disturbance in the functioning of, the mind or brain means that the person is unable to make a decision for herself. A person is deemed unable to make a decision when they cannot understand the information relevant to the decision, or retain that information, or use or weigh that information as part of the decision-making process, or communicate their decision. Two critical principles should be borne in mind. First, the fact that a woman has a mental health disorder, such as bipolar disorder, does not mean that she lacks capacity. A person who suffers from a mental health condition may very well be able to make decisions about their health. Second, simply because a woman might make an unwise or irrational decision, does not mean that she does not have capacity. In the abortion context, the courts have been willing to set a low bar for finding that women are competent to make their own choices. When it comes to decisions about childbirth, judges appear much readier to intervene.

In the highly publicised and controversial case of *Re AA*, a pregnant Italian woman with schizophrenia was sectioned and detained after suffering a mental breakdown during a visit to the UK. Some weeks before her due date, the National Health Service (NHS) trust providing her maternity care in detention approached the Court of Protection for an order authorising a caesarean section on the grounds that she had had two previous caesarean sections and there was consequently a risk of scar rupture should she give birth naturally. The court was not told, and apparently did not ask, whether the woman herself wished to have a vaginal birth or a repeat caesarean section. It accepted, without question, that the risk of scar rupture after two previous caesarean sections was sufficient to justify surgery. The court did not take account of, or consider the risks of surgery to the woman. Applying the 'best interests' principle, which permits the court to determine whether medical treatment is in an incapacitated person's best interest, the court authorised the caesarean section. The operation was duly performed and the baby taken into care. While the court recognised that the fetus did not have a separate, legally recognised right to life that could be wielded against its mother, the judge assumed that a woman's best interests are served by protecting her child from risk of harm. Subsequent cases have reached the same conclusion.

Midwifery evidence has been strikingly absent from decisions ordering caesarean section. In the case of *DD*, the woman in question was suffering from a number of mental health conditions. She had had five previous births. Her first three children were born by caesarean section and her most recent two children were born vaginally. The gestation of her current pregnancy was unknown. While the court undertook a careful analysis of the obstetric evidence, no midwifery evidence was presented to the court. The court authorised her forcible removal from her home, the administration of steroids in case the baby was delivered prematurely and a caesarean section. The woman had been willing to accept some ante-natal care and it is possible that a midwife could have established a relationship with her that would have helped see the pregnancy to term and avoided the need to use force to take her to hospital. Sadly, the focus on managing obstetric risks with obstetric solutions neglected the potential for a solution founded on the traditional, relational values of midwifery.

Informed consent and a right to evidence-based care

Consent to medical treatment would be a hollow principle without also recognising the preceding duty on the healthcare professional to provide information about the proposed treatment. Again, the principle is easy to state: the person must be told of the risks and benefits of a proposed medical intervention and the alternative choices that are available to her, including the choice to decline the intervention (see also Chapter 3). But informed consent is often overlooked in practice, particularly in maternity care when hospitals frequently provide partial information and consciously restrict women's options.

American lawyer Hermine Hayes Klein has proposed a three-stage process to assist caregivers in providing true informed consent in maternity care:

1. *Inform.* Tell the woman about what you observe to be going on at this moment in the pregnancy or birth. Tell her about all of the healthcare alternatives that are available to her. Not just the one you think she should do. Tell her as much as you know about the risks and benefits of each alternative, and what kind of evidence exists for this information. This part of the discussion should be a transfer of objective facts, and you should leave your opinion out of it.
2. *Advise.* Tell the woman what you think she should do. Tell her why. This is a good moment to express the limits of your own skills and knowledge. Are you advising a caesarean for breech because you haven't been trained in breech births? This is a time to mention that. This part of the discussion can be an expression of your subjective opinion about what you would counsel the woman to do.
3. *Support.* Support the woman in the exercise of a decision between the alternatives. This includes the decision not to follow your advice. It isn't informed consent unless the patient has the ability to choose an alternative other than the one that the provider recommends.

The first stage in the process of informed consent requires care providers to present women with the evidence that supports or undermines their recommended intervention. In effect, it imposes an obligation on healthcare professionals to provide evidence-based care and gives women a right to demand it. Critically, objective presentation of information demands honesty about the source of the evidence. Professionals should explain whether their recommendation is based on research evidence, expert opinion or clinical experience. In the case of a recommendation for amniotomy in a prolonged labour, for example, a care provider might be wise to explain that the Cochrane systematic review does not support amniotomy in prolonged labour, and that the recommendation is based on hospital policy and the professional's own clinical experience.

Assess your local maternity unit's information leaflet on induction. Does it provide adequate information to enable informed consent by a woman who is offered induction?

The final, supportive element of informed consent is particularly critical in maternity care when women must continue to be able to access healthcare for the birth and postnatal period. Women must be able to make a choice without fear that there will be adverse consequences for her care, such as additional, unnecessary procedures or even referral to social services, or that care will be withdrawn. If a woman consents to a procedure after coercive tactics have been used, it will be questionable whether she has given her true consent, and the healthcare professional may be at risk of liability for non-consented care. While civil claims for lack of consent have traditionally been difficult for women to bring on the grounds that the compensation for lack of consent will be low, increasing appreciation of the long-term traumatic effect of non-consented care in childbirth may make such claims more common.

Coercive behaviour by health professionals can include:

Warnings about the potential for the baby's death or disability that are not put into appropriate perspective using evidence and statistics.

Additional antenatal appointments for unnecessary tests and scans.

Pressure on other family members to influence the woman's decision.

Threat of referral to social services if the woman does not comply with a professional recommendation.

Withdrawal of care or refusal to make a referral to a supportive care provider.

When you are next working with women in their homes, clinics or hospital settings spend some time reflecting on the above and identify if you notice any of these behaviours.

Consent and the right to informed choice

While consent is at the centre of the legal understanding of the relationship between patient and care provider, it has significant limitations as the conceptual basis for patient choice. The very notion of 'consent' presupposes an affirmative answer. The question: 'Do you consent?' is inherently different from the question: 'Have you made a choice?'. A decision to refuse consent can be more difficult for a person to make and communicate than a decision to choose from a range of options. It would be more neutral to describe the process of obtaining consent as a process of informed decision making or informed choice.

The law has recognised a positive right to choice in childbirth. While the common law focuses on a traditional notion of consent, human rights law has developed a fuller appreciation of the right to make healthcare choices. In the UK, the Human Rights Act 1998 enshrines in law the rights in the European Convention on Human Rights. All state healthcare providers are obliged to respect the rights set out in the European Convention and a person can make a claim under the 1998 Act for a violation of their rights. Article 8 of the European Convention enshrines a right to private life, which has been interpreted by the European Court of Human Rights to include a woman's right to make decisions about childbirth. In *Ternovszky v Hungary*, the Court considered a claim by a woman who wished to give birth at home. She argued that the failure by the Hungarian state to regulate midwives so that they could attend homebirths meant that she had been denied her right to make choices about childbirth. The Court stated:

> 'Private life' is a broad term encompassing, inter alia, aspects of an individual's physical and social identity including the right to personal autonomy, personal development and to establish and develop relationships with other human beings and the outside world . . . and it incorporates the right to respect for both the decisions to become and not to become a parent . . . The notion of a freedom implies some measure of choice as to its exercise. The notion of personal autonomy is a fundamental principle underlying the interpretation of the guarantees of Article 8 . . . Therefore the right concerning the decision to become a parent includes the right of choosing the circumstances of becoming a parent. The Court is satisfied that the circumstances of giving birth incontestably form part of one's private life for the purposes of this provision.

Like the notion of consent, the right to choice is rooted in individual autonomy. But it recognises that choice sometimes requires positive support from others; it therefore offers much greater protection of autonomy than simple consent. In *Ternovszky*, the Court concluded that the state was obliged to provide a 'legal and institutional' environment that enabled women to make the choice to give birth outside hospital. This meant that midwives had to be properly regulated so that they could practice outside hospitals without fear of disciplinary sanctions. While the *Ternovszky* case concerned homebirth, the principle applies to all childbirth decisions – choice of birth partner, choice of position in labour, choice of pain relief and so on. A human rights-based approach provides a framework in which women can make choices and ensure that their choices are respected.

Observe a conversation between an obstetrician and/or midwife about a medical intervention. Is the woman given a choice? How is she supported if her choice differs from the professional recommendation?

As the Court noted in *Ternovszky*, Article 8 can be limited by reference to the rights of others, but compelling reasons would have to be advanced for any limitation. It is possible, for example, that a hospital could limit the number of birth partners that a woman has with her in hospital on the grounds of space. In the case of home birth, Article 8 gives the woman the right to choose to give birth at home, but the right might in theory be limited by risk to mother and baby. However, the traditional principle of consent would make it impossible to compel a competent woman to attend hospital and a midwife would be in breach of their professional obligations if they refused to provide care at home.

Respectful relationships

Informed consent is not an ethical panacea; it is neither the beginning nor the end of high-quality care. Rather, informed consent is an essential component of the broader principle of respectful care, namely care that respects a person's human dignity, which encompasses their right to humane treatment and treatment that promotes their autonomy. The starting point for good care is the relationship between woman and midwife or doctor. The relationship must be built on the principle of respect so that the process of informed decision making, which will occur multiple times over the course of a woman's care, can flourish. Consent that is given in the context of a disrespectful relationship is unlikely to be true consent.

A respectful relationship is particularly important in maternity care in part because the process of obtaining consent during childbirth can pose some significant practical difficulties. The pain and disorientation that women experience in childbirth is not always conducive to properly informed decision making. The woman is likely to rely heavily on her midwife or doctor to guide her decisions. If the midwife is discourteous, if she has failed to introduce herself, is physically rough or has spoken harshly, the woman's decisions will be tainted by disrespect. She may later reflect on her decisions and feel she did not give her real consent. As research shows, women who report negative emotions after their child's birth are more likely to have experienced poor relationships during labour. By contrast, women with good relationships with their caregivers during childbirth are more likely to have felt in control of decisions and to report positive experiences of labour.

Consider impediments to respectful maternity care and how these might be overcome.

Case studies

Maternity care suffers more acutely than many other areas of healthcare from the notion of 'routine' interventions, mandated by clinical policy and ingrained clinical practice that can sometimes appear impervious to advances in medical understanding. Two routine practices are discussed below with regard to the implications for informed consent.

When a woman is receiving intrapartum care, she will often experience a large number of minor physical interventions, such as palpation. Obtaining consent for each of these intrusions into the woman's space can be formalistic. It may be better to understand consent for minor physical interventions as part of an ongoing relationship between woman and midwife or doctor, in which the woman has agreed to the intrusion on an ongoing basis unless she withdraws her consent. However, the woman's agreement will be premised on a respectful relationship with her care provider, in which it is understood that interventions will be performed only when necessary and with due care.

Vaginal examinations

Vaginal examinations are a standard means of assessing women's progress in labour. While vaginal examinations are recognised as highly invasive and potentially painful, the fact that they are a standard part of midwifery practice often means that consent is not properly obtained.

Application to practice

The following example of a conversation between a woman and a midwife during the assessment of the woman prior to admission to the birth centre is illustrative:

Midwife: *You need to take your knickers off now and lie on the bed. I'm going to examine you.*

Woman: *I'd rather not be examined right now.*

Midwife: *I have to examine you to see how dilated you are.*

Woman: *I've been having contractions for ages, I really want to get into the birth centre and use the pool.*

Midwife: *We can't let you onto the birth centre unless you are 4 cm. I need to examine you.*

This is the first vaginal examination that the woman has experienced in labour. She is not initially given any information about why she needs an examination; the midwife assumes that she will comply with the request. Nor is she told what will happen during the examination, that the midwife will insert her fingers into the back of her vagina and feel her cervix. She is not told that it may be painful. She has not been informed of the risks of the examination and has not been offered any alternative, despite her request that the examination does not take place. When she is given an explanation for the necessity of the examination, it is based on hospital policy. While hospital policies do generally instruct midwives to perform an examination in order to assess cervical dilation before admission onto the labour ward or birth centre, vaginal examinations can never be compulsory, as consent must always be freely given.

Electronic fetal monitoring

In the UK, women experiencing 'high-risk' labours are routinely monitored by cardiotocography (CTG). The evidence for electronic fetal monitoring (EFM) is poor. The recent National Institute for Health and Care Excellence (NICE) draft intrapartum care guideline explained that there is very limited evidence that EFM improves outcomes for babies, interpretation of CTGs is prone to error and there is a high false positive rate. There are significant risks for the mother associated with EFM, including a significantly higher likelihood of an instrumental birth and caesarean section. It also makes it more likely that continuous one to one support by a midwife will not be provided during labour. Women are not generally informed of any of this information when they are placed on a monitor in labour (though they may have been told something of the problems with EFM in antenatal classes). They are not usually informed that they have a choice whether to accept continuous monitoring or that they can ask that the monitor is removed. The alternative – intermittent auscultation – is rarely offered, despite its benefits. In these circumstances, it is clear that women are not able to give informed consent to a practice that can have profound consequences for their experience of childbirth.

Conclusion

This chapter has explained the pre-eminent place of consent in medical ethics and the law. It has shown how that principle can be undermined in cases of mental incapacity and by routine practice during childbirth that does not give women the opportunity to explore alternative options for care. Women's autonomy is most fully protected by the twin rights to evidence-based care and informed choice. These rights provide a strong foundation for high-quality care in childbirth, but they can only be fully realised in the context of a respectful relationship between the woman and her care provider.

References

Airedale NHS Trust v Bland (1993) 12 BMLR 64.
Birthrights (2013) *The Dignity Survey 2013: Women's and Midwives' Experience of Dignity in Childbirth*, London: Birthrights. Available at: www.birthrights.org.uk.

Hayes Klein H. (2013) *Informed Consent in Childbirth*. Human Rights in Childbirth. Available at: http://humanrightsinchildbirth.com/informed-consent-in-childbirth/

HMSO (Her Majesty's Stationary Office) (2005) *Mental Capacity Act 2005*, London: HMSO.

Kitzinger S. (2005) *The Politics of Birth*, London: Elsevier.

National Institute for Health and Care Excellence (2014) *Intrapartum Care: Care of healthy women and their babies during childbirth – Draft for consultation*, London: NICE.

Nursing and Midwifery Council (2010) *Supporting Women in their Choice for Home Birth*, London: NMC.

Re AA [2013] EWCOP 4378.

Re MB (An Adult: Medical treatment) (1998) 40 BMLR 160.

Re SB [2013] EWCOP 1417.

Smyth R.M.D., Markham C., Dowswell T. (2013) *Amniotomy for Shortening Spontaneous Labour*, Cochrane Database of Systematic Reviews, Issue 6.

Stadylmayr W., Amsler F., Lemola S., et al. (2006) Memory of childbirth in the second year: the long-term effect of a negative birth experience and its modulation by the perceived intranatal relationship with caregivers. *Journal of Psychosomatic Obstetrics and Gynecology* 27(4): 211–224.

Stewart M. (2014) Vaginal examination: consent or coercion. Midwifery seminar, St Thomas' Hospital, 11 June 2014.

Ternovszky v Hungary [2010] ECHR 67545/09.

The Mental Health Trust v DD [2014] EWCOP 11.

Waldenstrom U., Hidingsson I., Rubertsson C., et al. (2004) A negative birth experience: prevalence and risk factors in a national sample. *Birth* 31(1):17–27.

8 Politics and birth

Patricia Lindsay

Aim

The aim of this chapter is to consider the influence of politics on healthcare provision, including maternity services, women's choices and how midwives work. It aims to stimulate the reader to engage with the political debate around maternity care, wherever we work and whatever we do. It also aims to debunk the myth that politics is the concern of a limited number of powerful elites who impose policies on a large constituency of powerless consumers. In other words, the chapter aims to show politics as it is – important, relevant and exciting.

Learning outcomes

By the end of this chapter the reader will be able to:

- Say what politics means in relation to healthcare
- Say how political decisions affect the provision of healthcare in the UK
- Identify areas of maternity care where political influences have had, or are having, an impact
- Understand the impact of political influences on midwifery, and its future as a distinct and autonomous profession
- Identify how they can engage with politics to make a difference to women's advocacy, birth choices and experiences
- Identify how political awareness can combat feelings of professional powerlessness

---

The comments in this chapter generally refer to healthcare in England, as Scotland, Wales and Northern Ireland may have slightly different political arrangements.

Introduction

Politics permeate every moment of our lives. It affects how we are born, how we live and how we die. When 'politics' is discussed the mental picture is often of politics with a capital P, that is, party politics, for example Conservative, Labour, Liberal Democrat, Scottish National Party (SNP), United Kingdom Independence Party (UKIP). Thoughts may then turn to what policies the parties espouse on health and maternity care, and whether or not we agree with them. Some of these thoughts will be based on our upbringing and possibly our personal views of social justice, developed through our experiences in childhood and adult life. Many people will have some party political affiliation but this may be viewed as one aspect of their lives or identity with limited relevance to their day-to-day experiences. Other people may not see how politics is relevant at all and would not think of themselves as political beings. This may partly be because the image of politics has perhaps become rather debased over the years. Politicians often get a bad press and political exposures ('sleaze') are hot sellers, especially of newspapers. This can be off-putting to the average person, who may have little patience with political scheming and would never dream of calling themselves 'political'. However anyone who has ever thought 'it's not fair', or who believes in equal rights for any apparently marginalised group has engaged with politics (Heywood, 2012). Politics is present in all our relationships (Tillett, 2011). We are, therefore, all political to some degree but the concepts are so much part of our everyday lives that we very often don't see them until they are threatened or challenged in some way. Politics is essentially about beliefs of how society should be run and what should be done to achieve the agreed goals.

A sprint through some political ideologies

This section aims to give a flavour of the key points of political ideologies, to help understand why politicians make the decisions they do. An ideology is, essentially, a coherent collection of beliefs about how society should be, how political power should be exercised to achieve the desired state and what action is needed. Thus each ideology proposes a different view of the ideal society, how it should be governed and a road map of how to achieve the vision. Some of the older ideologies were quite rigid but may now have lost a good deal of their force with increasing globalisation, the emergence of market economies in previously communist states and the emergence of variants on older themes such as 'New Labour'. Heywood (2012) identifies classical ideologies (Table 8.1) and those that are relatively new or emerging. It is worth thinking about some of these as they may help explain what beliefs drive the policies promulgated by the government of the day. They also help to explain what we see in the world around us. For example nationalism (or ethnic nationalism) has been a driving force behind the ethnic cleansing carried out by nationalist groups around the world. Britain has its own variant of nationalism, most obviously in the form of the National Front, although other groups espouse similar beliefs.

Newer ideologies include: feminism, multiculturalism, fundamentalism and ecologism. While none of the new ideologies is currently a powerful political force in the UK, the impact of some is felt in the actions and policies of the government in response to, for example, perceived threats to national security from groups that espouse fundamentalism.

Table 8.1 Classical ideologies

Label	Main Tenets	Variants
Conservatism	Tradition Natural social hierarchies Authoritarianism/paternalism Support for private ownership, for example of goods or wealth	New Right: return to family values Free-market economics More laissez-faire
Socialism	Equality and community Common ownership: the means of production and distribution are controlled by the state Support for welfare state Utopian vision	Communism Marxism-Leninism Social democracy/the Third Way
Liberalism	Freedom, justice and equality for all Individualism Limitations to state powers over the lives of individuals Reliance on market forces Meritocratic	Modern liberalism: greater acceptance of state intervention such as the welfare state
Nationalism	Views the nation as being the only legitimate form of political rule Self-determination Love of country	Ethnic nationalism
Fascism	Authoritarian nationalism, centred on a single charismatic leader Patriarchal Elitist	Neo-fascism
Anarchism	Unrestricted personal liberty Rejection and abolition of government and the law Social order will arise naturally	New anarchism Green anarchism – focuses on the environment

Source: Adapted from Haywood, 2012

In the UK we are essentially living in a capitalist society, which leans towards conservatism, socialism or liberalism, depending on which party (if any) has the overall majority in Parliament.

When healthcare professionals, including midwives, consider the influence of politics on their work it may produce feelings of resigned helplessness in the face of the government juggernaut, especially if the apparent choices are between accepting the status quo, leaving the profession or going on strike. However it does not have to be such a stark choice and midwives have several means of political engagement that will be clear by the end of the chapter. The next section reviews the context of healthcare and politics.

Healthcare provision and politics

Healthcare has always been a politicised phenomenon and nowadays is often seized upon as a rallying standard in party political elections. There are long-standing links between parliamentary politics and the National Health Service (NHS), stretching back to, and beyond, the launch of the NHS in 1948 as a free service, financed from taxes. Indeed there are sometimes accusations that the NHS is used as a political football, when patient expectations of more and better care are pitched against political demands for financial cutbacks (NHS Confederation, 2014). The government (Parliament) affects the NHS through legislation such as the Health and Social Care Act 2012, through standardisation and policies, such as those developed by the National Institute for Health and Care Excellence (NICE), and through targets, which may be set as a result of reports. Changes to NHS policy may be based on political expediency. An example of this is prescription charges, introduced in 1952 under a Conservative government, rescinded in 1965 under a Labour government but reintroduced in 1968 by the same government in response to rocketing NHS drug bills (NHS Choices, 2013; Politics.co.uk, 2014).

The political face of the NHS

The position of Secretary of State for Health is one of the most important in Parliament. He or she is the public face of government policy, responsible for driving through policy and accountable for the consequences. They need to be authoritative and show sympathy for the concerns of staff and the public about the NHS and how it is managed, while seeing that sometimes very unpopular changes are introduced. This can be risky to his or her career: the sacking of Andrew Lansley, the then Health Secretary, in 2012 by Prime Minister David Cameron was widely seen as damage limitation in the face of public uproar about the overhaul of the NHS. His successor, Jeremy Hunt, was said to have been chosen because he had a better 'bedside manner' than Lansley, but was judged to have less of an instinctive feel for the NHS (Burnham, quoted by Dabrowski, 2012).

Staff numbers are politically significant as staff pay costs are the biggest part of the NHS budget, 60 per cent for most NHS employers (DH, 2013). The next big political battlefield will be NHS pensions. The central NHS budget will also have an impact on skill mix and commissions for training places in nursing and midwifery. The future staffing of maternity care may see greater numbers of maternity support workers and doulas taking over work such as labour support, which has traditionally been done by midwives (King's Fund, 2011). This would be a politically astute move as it would increase client satisfaction while reducing staff costs. Furthermore the King's Fund report (2011) argues that there is little evidence for a correlation between staffing levels and maternity outcomes.

Des Jardin (2001), writing about nursing in the United States (US), notes that government decisions influence the clinical work environment through legislation, rates of pay, resource allocation and structural reform. She further notes that many (US) nurses see no relation between their working conditions and their own political apathy. The same may well be true of midwives in the UK.

Politics, policy and reports

Government interest in healthcare and health provision is acute, and rightly so as the government is responsible for paying for most of it, from money raised though our taxes. There is a need to monitor provision and expenditure to try to ensure that basic needs are provided for at the lowest possible cost. Thus healthcare came to be seen as a business and management had to be slick and efficient. Early attempts at achieving this were seen in the managerialist approach in the late twentieth century, starting with the Griffiths reforms, detouring round Thatcher's purchaser/provider split, with the most recent (at the time of publication) being Lansley's reforms initially set out in the White Paper *Equity and Excellence: Liberating the NHS* (DH, 2010). Recent criticisms have centred on the perception that these reforms are privatisation by stealth, while fundamental issues such as quality and caring for an increasingly aged patient group are ignored. While these charges are hotly denied, it is interesting that Chapter 2 of the Health and Social Act (2012) is about competition (Smith, 2014).

It could also be argued that recent attempts at restructuring are merely tinkering with the edges of a much bigger problem. It is axiomatic that government policy can affect the income of the electorate through taxation and benefits freezes. The recent period of austerity has affected those on low incomes disproportionately and deepened income inequalities (Joseph Rowntree Foundation, 2014). It has long been accepted that an individual's socioeconomic circumstances have a profound impact on their health and some public health provision, including the current Healthy Child Programme, has been based on this understanding (Blair and Maccauley, 2013; DH 2009). However not all reports linking health outcomes to social circumstances have been warmly welcomed. An example of this is the Black report (Townsend et al., 1988). Commissioned by a Labour government, it was the report of an expert committee chaired by Sir Douglas Black, and it identified economic inequality as the biggest determinant of health outcomes. By the date of publication a Conservative government was in power. The publication date for this politically sensitive report was arranged for the August Bank Holiday weekend in 1980, with only 260 copies available. This was widely seen as an attempt at suppression because the recommendations to tackle poverty, especially child poverty, were seen as too expensive. This political attitude matters to midwives because women may be more exposed to the impact of poverty, including poor living conditions, than men (Women's Budget Group, 2012). A woman with a young child, or children, may be less able to escape the domestic environment, which may be crowded, damp, dirty or infested, by going to work. Women also take much, if not most, of the responsibility for producing and raising the next generation. The expectation is that the offspring will be healthy but this will not be the case if the woman is struggling with social and economic inequalities that limit her ability to make healthy choices.

Healthcare has been the subject of numerous reports commissioned by the House of Commons. In 2003 a House of Commons health committee reported on maternity services (Hinchliffe, 2003). Points of concern raised were the high caesarean section rate, which was 25.5 per cent in 2012–2013 (NCT, 2013), lack of continuity of care and one to one care in labour, and gaps in skills mix in maternity care. More than ten years on we are still dealing with these problems. Shribman (2007) authored a report on service reconfiguration in maternity. The same concerns about high rates of intervention were highlighted and solutions proposed included greater centralisation of obstetric services, supported by midwife-led units. This was not well received in some areas and public protests at closure of local services were well publicised. There were political debates and questions in the House of Commons as a result (Hansard, 2010).

The current state of maternity care has been the subject of activism by national groups such as the National Federation of Women's Institutes (NFWI), who, with the National Childbirth trust (NCT), produced a report (NFWI and NCT, 2013) on women's experiences of maternity care. Sadly this highlighted the same issues of lack of continuity of care and poor postnatal support affecting women's care in childbirth as had been reported before.

NHS reforms in the early twenty-first century

Following the passing of the Health and Social Care Act 2012 a series of reforms started. Service planning needs were part of the new arrangements, directed by a politically independent NHS commissioning board and policed by Monitor, a health-specific economic regulator (Nuffield Trust, 2014). All trusts would have foundation status. As the aim was to devolve power from central government, clinical commissioning groups (CCGs) were set up to commission local health services. They have responsibility for using 60 per cent of the NHS budget and are accountable to the secretary of state for health. These general practitioner (GP)-led groups are responsible for identifying and meeting the healthcare needs in the local area. The groups consist of GPs, lay members, a secondary (i.e. specialist) consultant and a nurse. Figure 8.1 provides an overview of the NHS structure in England following reform.

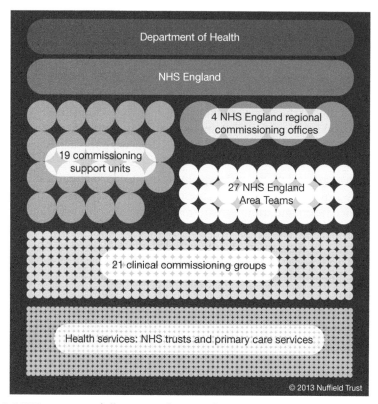

Figure 8.1 NHS structure following reforms, after April 2013

Source: Copyright Nuffield Trust, 2013

A joint statement offering advice on commissioning maternity services was issued by the NCT, RCM (Royal College of Midwives) and RCOG (Royal College of Obstetricians) in 2013 (NCT et al., no date). There are 211 CCGs in England at the time of writing. The CCGs work with local authorities through health and well-being boards. Commissioning support units (CSUs) provide CCGs with infrastructure support such as data management, finance and contracting. The CSUs will become private companies in 2015. This 'privatisation' has been seen as part of a wider fragmentation of NHS services and arguably reflects the underlying political ideology to the changes. For example, where previously a foundation trust could only raise 2–4 per cent of its income by treating private (paying) patients, under the new provisions this cap will potentially rise to 49 per cent of total income (RCN, no date).

Trigger

Watch this short presentation on the new NHS:

http://www.kingsfund.org.uk/projects/nhs-65/alternative-guide-new-nhs-england

Is it clear where maternity services sit in the new structure? Find out who is responsible for commissioning maternity services in your area.

The Department of Health provides £4.9 billion per year for medical and professional training (King's Fund, 2013a). However responsibility for educating the healthcare workforce rests with local education and training boards (LETBs), of which there are 13 in England. They are responsible to the Department of Health through Health Education England. Each LETB works with stakeholders such as deaneries, health service providers and education providers such as universities to make sure that local workforce needs are met. This is set out in Figure 8.2.

In the wake of the care failings at the Mid-Staffordshire NHS Foundation Trust, reported by Francis (2013), quality of care has become a major part of the government agenda for health. The Care Quality Commission (CQC) has produced a consultation document on proposed changes to how it regulates, inspects and monitors care (CQC, 2013). This was partly in response to a Commons Health Committee (2011) report that outlined CQC failings in setting priorities and meeting objectives.

However the King's Fund response indicates some concerns about how workable some of the proposals are and whether the CQC is actually resourced to meet its own targets set out in this document (King's Fund, 2013b). Figure 8.3 indicates how providers are regulated.

It should be noted that the function of Monitor changed with the Health and Social Care Act 2012. Prior to this Act its function had been largely assessing, monitoring and regulating foundation trusts. Since the introduction of the Act the remit has been broadened to include financial leadership and quality of services. It works collaboratively with the CQC but does not carry out spot checks.

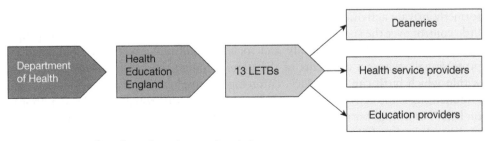

Figure 8.2 Funding for education and training

Source: Adapted from King's Fund, 2013a

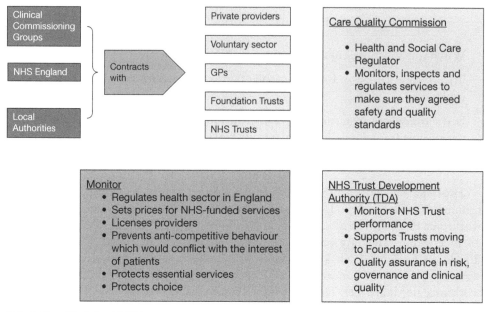

(Adapted from King's Fund 2013a)

Figure 8.3 The regulation of providers in the new NHS in England

Source: Adapted from King's Fund, 2013a

The strengthening of regulatory oversight is one outcome of the Francis report (Francis, 2013). However there seems to be some overlap between the functions of the three monitoring bodies, CQC, Monitor and TDA (NHS Trust Devlopment Authority), which opens up questions about scope of action, potential for conflict and the potential for gaps in oversight of services. A statement of intent issued by the government goes some way to explaining how these bodies will work together (Monitor et al., no date).

Political control and women's health choices

As Chapter 5 discusses, it can be argued that the state has now assumed control over events such as birth and death. The move from home to hospital birth has ensured that formerly private activities are now played out in public spaces where the woman has little control over the space she occupies, the people who accompany her or the people who care for her. These culturally and socially significant events are dominated by professionals, who act as agents of the state, dictating the conditions or boundaries within which birth can take place, enforcing the application of policies of care and criminalising some activities. For example, in 2014 a case brought by a local authority on behalf of a child born with fetal alcohol syndrome was allowed to go to the Court of Appeal, having failed at an initial hearing. The allegation was that the mother's excessive alcohol intake in pregnancy constituted the offence of poisoning. This has raised questions about the legal rights of the fetus. The Court of Appeal rejected the claim. However this does not preclude a future claim and if this is successful it may alter the legal status of the fetus and make it possible to criminalise maternal behaviour in pregnancy. This would require legislation and the political will to exert greater control over childbearing women.

Application to practice

Helen, a para 5 and 16 weeks pregnant, is a woman in your caseload. Her previous children are all in care as she has persistently misused alcohol over many years. What resources are available to you to help her control her alcohol use?

State control over midwifery has been apparent in the recent requirement, following the Scott report (2010) and the European Union (EU) directive on cross-border healthcare (EU, 2011), that, from July 2014, all nurses and midwives must declare that they have indemnity insurance in order to maintain their registration (NMC, 2014). This was therefore a political decision that will have a profound impact on midwives' work and women's choices. Midwives who do not have or cannot afford indemnity cover are effectively barred from practising. The greatest impact is likely to be felt by independent midwives who may be unable to practice. This statutory requirement effectively makes the NHS and private/independent hospitals monopoly providers of maternity care, unless independent midwives group together to set up small businesses or social enterprises. The Law Commission report (2014) comments that any special rules for independent midwives must be a matter for government (Law Commission, 2014). This is one area where effective political engagement by midwives can have an impact.

This report and draft bill produced by the Law Commission (2014) makes provision for a single legal framework for all healthcare regulatory bodies, including the NMC. If enacted it may make it possible for regulatory bodies to investigate poor practice proactively and may also bring changes for supervision of midwives.

Political influences affect the way medical and midwifery staff are socialised into their roles, the hierarchical structure of healthcare services and medicalisation of women's health. These in turn affect power relations in maternity care (Tillett, 2011). This includes consent and informed choice, and who has the last word when decisions about birth are made. For example, while consumerism is acknowledged by the routine use of birth plans and offering 'choices' for care, the options often appear as a limited list that is preselected by the maternity service. Occasionally choices are denied if the needs of the service conflict with the woman's wishes. One such area is the choice to birth at home, which may be withdrawn if the service cannot provide the midwives to attend. The underlying issue here is resource allocation: when money is tight it may be spent on services that meet government targets or that may attract external funding such as 'cutting-edge' innovations. Intensive care facilities or the pioneering of new and exciting surgical techniques will attract money because they are headline grabbing and 'sexy'; normal childbirth is not. Breast feeding is definitely not.

Have a look at this short film *Why birth matters – #feministbirth*:

https://m.youtube.com/watch?v=rTJKS3zNN9Y

One of the participants says that birth is political. Is birth political and if so, why?

Women wanting an option that is not part of routine provision may be denied, such as those wanting a home water-birth after a previous caesarean section. Most obstetricians would not agree to this and it may be hard for women to argue their case in an encounter where they may have very little power. This is an interesting situation since, as the law currently stands, the woman has a right to give birth where she wants to and only in specific circumstances, such as a court order, can anyone stop her. However, to avoid being labelled as awkward, the politics of conformity may lead to her accepting what is offered rather than what she feels is right for her. She also has the legal right to choose who attends the birth. She may choose to birth without professional attendants: free birthing has become a hot topic and there is some confusion about whether or not it is legal. It is, as long as an unqualified person does not take responsibility for the woman's care (NMC, 2013). There is also the issue of social congruence between doctor and 'patient': if the woman does not share the same cultural and intellectual background as the obstetrician she may find it hard to express her needs, or argue her case, and she may not get a hearing if she does. The midwife, however, may be seen as having more social congruence and less distance from the woman. This may make it easier for the woman to challenge the midwife or ask questions about her care.

Kerri is 43 weeks pregnant and attending an antenatal clinic in the hospital. She has been told to lie on her back and take her knickers off as she will need a vaginal examination. A doctor (who she has never met before) is standing over her, telling her that policy dictates that she must have labour induced. You know she doesn't want this. You have explained the risk of post-dates pregnancy but she is adamant. National and local policy and risk aversion are controlling this conversation. How powerful do you think she feels? What can you as a midwife do to enable her to express her wishes and achieve her goal of a natural, spontaneous birth?

In the above scenario (which will, no doubt, be familiar to a number of readers) the medical professional might be sympathetic, or might adopt a position of intellectual dominance, by the assumption of superior knowledge. Equally, the position may be one of moral dominance, by pointing out the potential harm to the fetus (shroud-waving). The merits of Kerri's request could be the subject of endless debate. However there is no doubt that the underlying structures that have led to this situation are political.

The impact of political decisions on midwives' work and care of women

Some of the impact results from decisions to standardise healthcare, embodied in national policy documents such as NICE guidelines. These are not mandatory but few trusts (and few midwives) would risk ignoring them.

Budget allocation and resources are another area that is affected by political decisions. This may be something major such as the closure of a free-standing unit to save money. It may be less high profile, such as the substitution of one (useful and effective) drug for another, cheaper and less effective option. Services may be cut back, for example, postnatal visits or parent education classes. Staffing shortfalls are common, with midwifery workforce requirements often estimated at levels below those required for the level of activity and acuity. This has a direct effect on whether women get one to one care in labour. This in turn affects satisfaction for women and midwives. Some trusts use support workers and doulas to fill the gap but this does not address the need for care that is provided by a registered (and accountable) midwife. Specialist midwife posts may be cut, or left unfilled, as a result of budget pressures, leaving often very vulnerable women exposed to risk. Sure Start centres were part of a strategy to provide support for women and families with particular support needs. However, budget cuts since 2011 have resulted in withdrawal of facilities, such as on-site childcare, from many and the introduction of charges for services in some areas (4children, 2012).

Trigger

Think about a situation where you felt that political influences had affected the resources available to you when caring for women. Write down what resources were affected. These may have been material, such as equipment, structural such as changes to the way the maternity service was provided to women or staffing/skill mix.

Why do you think these changes were successful?

The childbirth care needs of the dispossessed

Some groups of women have particular maternity care needs that are not always met. These are often women on the fringes of society and invisible to many. They include women prisoners, trafficked women, asylum seekers and the homeless. A House of Commons report (2003) noted that some women had difficulty accessing maternity services and, once in the system, may not have received appropriate care, because the system is set up to cater for the needs of English-speaking and culturally competent women, who have access to GP services, and who understand how the system works. Political awareness and advocacy on the part of midwives could do much to remedy this service deficit for the disadvantaged. In the meantime it is often left to campaigners such as Sheila Kitzinger (Kitzinger, 2005) or charities such as the Eaves Poppy Project (Eaves, 2014) to plug the gap.

Trigger

Find out what care provision your local maternity service makes for women who could be considered to be dispossessed. This may include women who are refugees, asylum seekers, homeless or trafficked women.

If this is not seen as a problem in your area speak to a charity such as St Mungo's or the Salvation Army about what they do.

Conclusion

In autumn 2014, for the first time in its history, members of the RCM took industrial action. This was largely about midwives' pay. However, when attention is paid to other issues such as health outcomes, especially for poor or marginalised women, it is clear that political awareness and activism by midwives is essential. This may not be easy: tiredness, work-related stress and the complexity of political processes can all lead to apathy. However political awareness by midwives:

- Guards women by ensuring they can exercise true choice about their care
- Guards women and families by fighting for the resources needed for excellent care
- Ensures that the physical and psychological health of women and families is a fundamental and non-negotiable right, not merely a desirable outcome
- Helps protect women from discrimination
- Protects women's rights
- Protects the midwifery profession's right to practice as midwives.

Engagement with policy makers may be difficult but it may reap rewards for women and midwives. It is also essential to build links with consumer groups: alliances with groups who represent the interests of women make any actions more likely to succeed. Political action can be taken through:

- Professional organisations such as RCM or the Royal College of Nursing Midwifery Forum

- Political groups such as the Association for Improvements in Maternity Care (AIMS) or the NCT
- Finding out about meetings of the All Party Parliamentary group on Maternity (APPG). These are often open to the public
- Accessing electronic information for example through the Department of Health website and the Policy Studies website
- Contacting your member of parliament
- Voting: you cannot reasonably complain about government policy if you couldn't be bothered to vote.

Make sure that anything you choose to do is legal and does not jeopardise your registration.

Midwives' roles were diminished over the last century not because of their failure as caregivers but because of their failure to respond to the political challenges they faced. There are many understandable reasons for this behaviour in the past, but to repeat it would be folly.

(Declercq, 1994, p. 237)

References

4children (2012) 4children's 2012 census of Sure Start Centres. Online at: http://www.4children.org.uk/News/Detail/4Childrens-2012-Census-of-Childrens-Centres

Blair M. and Maccauley C. (2013) *The Healthy Child Programme: How did we get here and where should we go?* Paediatrics and Child Health seminar. Online at: http://www.ihv.org.uk/uploads/HCP%20how%20did%20we%20get%20here%20and%20where%20should%20we%20go.pdf

CQC (Care Quality Commission) (2013) *A New Start* London: Care Quality Commission. Online at: http://www.cqc.org.uk/sites/default/files/documents/cqc_consultation_2013_tagged_0.pdf

Commons Health Committee (2011) *Annual Accountability Hearing with the Care Quality Commission*, 9th Report. Online at: http://www.publications.parliament.uk/pa/cm201012/cmselect/cmhealth/1430/143002.htm

Dabrowski R. (2012) Facing the future: What will the NHS look like under Hunt? *Midwives* 6: 38–40

Declercq E. (1994) A cross-national analysis of midwifery politics: 6 lessons for midwives. *Midwifery* 10(4): 232–237

Des Jardin K (2001) Political involvement in nursing: education and empowerment. *AORN Journal* 74(4): 468–475

DH (Department of Health) (2009) *Healthy Child Programme: Pregnancy and the first 5 years*. London: Department of Health. Online at: https://www.gov.uk/government/uploads/system/uploads/attachment_data/file/167998/Health_Child_Programme.pdf

DH (2010) *Equity and Excellence: Liberating the NHS*. London: Department of Health. Online at: https://www.gov.uk/government/uploads/system/uploads/attachment_data/file/213823/dh_117794.pdf

DH (2013) *NHS Pay Review Body Review for 2014, written evidence from the Health Department for England September 2013*. London: Department of Health. Online at: https://www.gov.uk/government/uploads/system/uploads/attachment_data/file/284630/NHSPRB_Written_Evidence_2014-_Final_Version.pdf

Eaves (2014) *The Poppy Project* . Eaves: London. Online at: http://www.eavesforwomen.org.uk/about-eaves/our-projects/the-poppy-project

European Union (2011) *Directive 2011/24/EU of the European Parliament and of the Council of 9 March 2011 on the application of patients' rights in cross-border healthcare.* Online at: http://eur-lex.europa.eu/LexUriServ/LexUriServ.do?uri=OJ:L:2011:088:0045:0065:en:PDF

Francis R. (2013) *Report of the Mid-Staffordshire NHS Foundation Trust Public Inquiry.* Online: http://www.midstaffspublicinquiry.com/report

Hansard (2010) *House of Commons Official Report: Parliamentary Debates (Hansard) 29 June 2010 512(23).* London: House of Commons. Online at: http://www.publications.parliament.uk/pa/cm201011/cmhansrd/chan23.pdf

Heywood A (2012) *Political Ideologies.* Basingstoke: Palgrave Macmillan.

Hinchliffe D. (2003) *Provision of Maternity Services: Fourth Report of Session 2002–2003.* London: House of Commons Health Committee. Online at: http://www.publications.parliament.uk/pa/cm200203/cmselect/cmhealth/464/464.pdf

House of Commons (2003) *Inequalities in Access to Maternity Services: Eighth Report of Session 2002–2003.* London: House of Commons. Online at: http://www.parliament.the-stationery-office.co.uk/pa/cm200203/cmselect/cmhealth/696/696.pdf

Joseph Rowntree Foundation (2014) *Is Austerity Having a Disproportionate Effect on the Poorest people?* Joseph Rowntree Foundation. Online at: http://www.jrf.org.uk/austerity-bristol

King's Fund (2011) *Staffing in Maternity Units.* London: The King's Fund. Online at: http://www.kingsfund.org.uk/sites/files/kf/Staffing_in_maternity_units_Kings_Fund_March2011.pdf

King's Fund (2013a) *How is the New NHS Structured?* London: King's Fund. Online at: http://www.kingsfund.org.uk/audio-video/how-new-nhs-structured

King's Fund (2013b) *Consultation Response: A New Start – consultation on changes to the way the CQC regulates, inspects and monitors care.* London The King's Fund. Online at: http://www.kingsfund.org.uk/sites/files/kf/field/field_publication_file/consultation-cqc-regulate-inspect-monitor-care-aug13.pdf

Kitzinger S. (2005) *The Politics of Birth.* London: Elsevier

Law Commission (2014) *Regulation of Health Care Professionals; Regulation of Social Care Professionals in England.* Online at: http://lawcommission.justice.gov.uk/docs/lc345_regulation_of_healthcare_professionals.pdf

Monitor, CQC (Care Quality Commission) and TDA (Trust Development Authority) (no date) *How Monitor, the Care Quality Commission and the NHS Trust Development Authority will work together to assess how well-led organisations are.* Online at: https://www.gov.uk/government/uploads/system/uploads/attachment_data/file/312990/Well-led_framework_statement_of_intent_1_.pdf

NCT (National Childbirth Trust) (2013) *Maternity Statistics.* Online at http://www.nct.org.uk/professional/research/maternity%20statistics/maternity-statistics-england

NCT, RCM and RCOG (National Childbirth Trust, Royal Collage of Midwives and Royal College of Obstetricians and Gynaecologists) (no date) Making Sense of Commissioning Maternity Services in England: Some issues for Clinical Commissioning Groups to consider. Online at: https://www.rcm.org.uk/sites/default/files/Advice%20to%20CCGs%20final%20version.pdf

NFWI (National Federation of Women's Institutes) and NCT (2013) *Support Overdue: Women's experiences of maternity services.* London: National Federation of Women's

Institutes and the National Childbirth Trust. Online at: http://www.thewi.org.uk/__data/assets/pdf_file/0006/49857/support-overdue-final-15-may-2013.pdf

NHS Choices (2013) *The History of the NHS in England.* Online at: http://www.nhs.uk/NHSEngland/thenhs/nhshistory/Pages/NHShistory1948.aspx

NHS Confederation (2014) *Two Sides of the Same Coin*, April, Issue 271. Online at: http://www.nhsconfed.org/resources/2014/04/two-sides-of-the-same-coin-balancing-quality-and-finance-to-deliver-greater

NMC (Nursing and Midwifery Council) (2013) *Free Birthing.* London: Nursing and Midwifery Council. Online at: http://www.nmc-uk.org/Nurses-and-midwives/Regulation-in-practice/Regulation-in-Practice-Topics/Free-birthing1/

NMC (2014) *Professional Indemnity Arrangement: A new requirement for registration.* London: Nursing and Midwifery Council. Online at: http://www.nmc-uk.org/Documents/Registration/PII/PII%20final%20guidance.pdf

Nuffield Trust (2013) *Slideshow: The new NHS in England: Structure and Accountability.* Online at: http://www.nuffieldtrust.org.uk/our-work/projects/coalition-governments-health-and-social-care-reforms

Nuffield Trust (2014) *The Coalition Government's Health and Social Care Reforms.* Online at: http://www.nuffieldtrust.org.uk/our-work/projects/coalition-governments-health-and-social-care-reforms

Politics.co.uk (2014) *NHS Prescription Charges.* Online at: http://www.politics.co.uk/reference/nhs-prescription-charges

RCN (Royal College of Nursing) (no date) *What Does the Health and Social Care Act mean?* London: Royal College of Nursing. Online at: http://www.rcn.org.uk/__data/assets/pdf_file/0008/461798/HSCA_FINAL.pdf

Scott F. (2010) *Independent Review of the Requirement to have Insurance or Indemnity as a Condition of Registration as a Healthcare Professional.* London: Department of Health. Online at: https://www.gov.uk/government/publications/independent-review-of-the-requirement-to-have-insurance-or-indemnity-as-a-condition-of-registration-as-a-healthcare-professional

Shribman C. (2007) *Making it Better: For Mother and Baby.* London: Department of Health. Online at: http://webarchive.nationalarchives.gov.uk/20080814090357/dh.gov.uk/en/Publicationsandstatistics/Publications/PublicationsPolicyAndGuidance/DH_065053

Smith J. (2014) Politics: A matter for midwives? *British Journal of Midwifery* 22(5): 312

Tillett J. (2011) Politics, power and birth. *J. Perinat. Neonat. Nurs.* 25(2): 108–110

Townsend P., Davidson N. and Whitehead M. (1988) *Inequalities in Health: The Black Report and The Health Divide.* London: Penguin

UK government (2012) *Health and Social Care Act.* Online at: http://www.legislation.gov.uk/ukpga/2012/7/pdfs/ukpga_20120007_en.pdf?utm_source=UKHF ailing+list&utm_campaign=8fef7ceaff-UKHF_themed_briefing_Health_inequalities2_28_2014&utm_medium=email&utm_term=0_a21eedeaeb-8fef7ceaff-284936601

Women's Budget Group (2012) *The Impact on Women of the Budget 2012.* Online at: http://wbg.org.uk/pdfs/The-Impact-on-Women-of-the-Budget-2012-FINAL.pdf

<table>
<tr><td>9</td><td></td></tr>
</table>

Social policy for midwives

Mandie Scamell and
Andy Alaszewski

Aim

The aim of this chapter is to examine the nature of social policy making in contemporary government and its impact on midwifery practice.

Learning outcomes

By the end of this chapter the reader will be able to:

- Identify some of the key maternity policy reforms
- Discuss the ways policy shapes maternity services and current midwifery practice
- Understand the importance of the critical analysis of social policy
- Begin to critically evaluate contemporary maternity policy
- Explain how your own practice is influenced by social policy

---

Introduction

This chapter provides readers with the opportunity to engage with some of the key debates within the policy literature related to the practice of midwifery. Through description and analysis of the expansion of the state's interest in pregnancy and childbirth, the current health policy context of the maternity services and the centrality of risk within contemporary health policy, readers are encouraged to critically evaluate their role in birth management practices in the United Kingdom. The chapter begins with a description of the origins of health policy within the wider political framework of liberal reform. An analysis of maternity policy in relation to the medicalisation of childbirth project follows this description. Finally, the chapter moves on to critically evaluate the impact of the contemporary policy emphasis on informed choice and risk management.

What is health policy?

Among the diverse and disparate definitions of social/health policy that can be found in the literature, some are quite complex and others simple (Howlett et al., 1995). Despite this apparent struggle to pin down what is meant by social/health policy, or perhaps because of it, the everyday meaning of policy, that is how policy is understood by practitioners in their everyday practice is generally taken as a given (Alaszewski and Brown, 2012). This means that those of us tasked with enacting upon policy publications in our everyday care of women and their families are more concerned with the practical tasks of 'making it happen' rather than the pondering upon what it actually is. This approach to social policy, though pragmatic, tends to provoke compliance without enquiry, critique or question. This chapter discusses maternity care within the maternity policy context, with the opportunity to reflect more abstractly upon what social policy is and how it shapes the way we deliver maternity care services. By capturing the key components of the current academic critique of social policy and policy making, this chapter aims to engender a more reflective and analytical approach to policy interpretation.

The development of policy making

Broadly speaking, policy can be understood as the bureaucratic means through which governments in contemporary society seek to protect citizens from misfortunes such as disease and poverty. In this chapter we focus on the ways in which ideas about what governments should do provide the context for midwifery practice. Readers who want a more detailed analysis of the policy-making processes that connect ideas to action can find these in texts that focus on policy making (see for example Alaszewski and Brown, 2012; Hill, 2013).

The roots of social policy can be traced back to the nineteenth century when social reformers identified social problems that the state could and should deal with. For example Jeremy Bentham (1748–1832), the utilitarian philosopher developed plans for the rational management of poverty and crime based on model workhouses and prisons. During this period reformers and their various campaigns had some success in persuading a reluctant state to take on responsibility for the wellbeing of vulnerable individuals. The emerging social reforms of this period were generally seen as progressive reforms that laid the foundation for the development of the welfare state in the mid-twentieth century (see Box 9.1). However, there were some aspects of the reforms

---

Box 9.1   Key points for historic development of health policy: State expansion and the development of social policy

- At the start of the nineteenth century the role of the state was limited mainly to the defense of the realm and the maintenance of law and order

(continued)

(continued)

- In the nineteenth century there was a reluctant expansion of the scope of the state as reformers identified social problems that the state could and should address
- In the early twentieth century there was a rapid and relatively enthusiastic expansion of state activities that culminated in the formation of the welfare state

that are now seen as less benign. It is this more discerning approach to policy that offers the reflective practitioner the tools necessary to critically evaluate their own role in relation to current health policy agendas.

Health policy and childbearing

Health policy emerged as a distinct area of public policy-making activity as the government involvement in healthcare provision intensified in the middle of the last century (Alaszewski and Brown, 2012). With the post-war formation of the National Health Service (NHS) in 1948, health policy became both a well-defined and integral part of the government's efforts to invest in and plan public services.

Until the end of the nineteenth century, the expansion of state involvement had limited impact on childbirth and midwifery but this changed with the Liberal reforms of the early twentieth century. As child rearing, pregnancy and childbirth became a focus of health policy, so the state needed experts who would be willing and able to manage the problem on its behalf. For the supervision of pregnancy and childbirth the state reshaped an established occupation, midwifery. The Midwives Act (1902) established a national regulatory authority, the Central Midwives Board, consisting mainly of male physicians and surgeons. The Act specified that from 1905 'No woman shall habitually and for gain attend women in childbirth unless she be certified under this Act' (Clause 1 Section 1).

Trigger

Locate the Nursing and Midwifery Council website.

From the landing page explore how to find professional regulation documents.

Identify which of the regulation documents apply to the practice of a student midwife.

While state registration can be seen as a benevolent development, ensuring the safety of mothers and their children through the provision of qualified and supervised midwives, it can also be seen as representing a major shift in the nature of childbirth. Women were no longer free to choose their own birth attendant but had to have one who was trained and supervised by medical experts. For Katz Rothman this marks a shift from birth as a process that the pregnant woman controlled to birth as a medical event in which pregnancy is defined as 'a problem of medical management . . . a site of screening and diagnosis at all times for all purposes' (Katz Rothman, 2014, p. 2).

Application to practice

Whether or not midwives are aware of it, what we do, how we do it and why we do it is shaped by social policy. Thus the 1902 Midwives Registration Act recast midwives as agents of the state who had to apply medical knowledge to a medicalised process and report the outcomes to medical authorities. As Katz Rothman (2014) notes, this medicalisation of both midwifery and childbirth endures but many fail to notice it as it is so taken-for-granted and engrained into midwifery practice.

Maternity policy in context

Maternity care policy is not made in isolation. Instead it should be understood as being part of a wider political and policy context. The maternity health policy agenda over the last 25 years echoes a wider and unprecedented shift towards centering the patient in both healthcare provision and health policy (Giddens, 1998). Public/patient consultation and verification has not only been sought in issues of direct care, but also in the policy-making process itself, privileging both patient choice and expert patient initiatives (Alaszewski, 2007).

A central component of contemporary maternity policy is user involvement and women's informed choice. For example the Department of Health's policy document *Maternity Matters* (2007, p. 17) set out a national choice guarantee 'as a way to drive the essential improvements in the quality, safety and accessibility of service'.

Trigger

Maternity Matters is an important maternal health policy document. Locate this document from the National Archives. Identify the national choice guarantee.

Do you think the Trust you currently work in complies with this policy document?

The active endorsement of women-centered care and informed choice in contemporary maternity policy encourages women to reflect upon their pregnant bodies, adjust their lifestyle, optimise the health of their unborn child and purposefully design or plan their birth experience (Lupton, 1999, pp. 59– 85). Evidence of this self-regulation and planning in pregnancy is demonstrated in the plethora of pregnancy and birth texts available. See for example Marshall and Woollett's critique of pregnancy texts in *Fit to Reproduce? The Regulative Role of Pregnancy Texts* (2000). With the emphasis on informed choice, every pregnant woman is seen as being responsible for ensuring that they give birth to and nurture a healthy baby. Thus mothers have to demonstrate to midwives, health visitors and others that they are, 'good mothers' who are both healthy and competent of making sensible decisions. The term – good mother – is highlighted here in inverted commas because as the academic analysis of motherhood has demonstrated, the meaning of what it is to be a good mother should never be taken as a given. What constitutes a good mother changes over time and place. In other words, how mothers should behave is in part at least, socially constructed. Furthermore, the term good mother is never neutral. Ideas around good mothering that drive midwifery public health interventions, such as smoking cessation and breast feeding promotion, can and do instill feelings of inadequacy, guilt and even shame if women fail to live up to expectations set down by midwives (this idea is explored below in relation to pregnant drug takers).

Trigger

To strengthen understanding of the concept of good motherhood you are advised to read the following:

- *Being a 'good mother': Managing breastfeeding and merging identities* by Marshall and Woollett. 2000
- *'The best thing for the baby': Mothers' concepts and experiences related to promoting their infants' health and development'* by Lupton. 1999

Application to practice

We recommend that you consider this practice exercise before reading the rest of the chapter to enhance your understanding. Read the scenario below and consider the numbered points listed at the bottom of this section.

Emma is attending your antenatal clinic at 28 weeks gestation and is expecting her second baby. At booking Emma informed you that she was smoking around 20 cigarettes a day. You offered to refer Emma to the Cessation of Smoking Support Programme as per local protocol but Emma assured you that she managed to give up smoking easily last time she was pregnant and that she did not need any extra support.

As Emma reclines on the examination couch you notice that she smells of cigarette smoke. Emma requests that you listen into the baby's heart rate and as you do you observe fetal tachycardia consistent with maternal smoking.

When you offer to discuss with Emma the benefits of giving up smoking she responds: 'Oh that's okay, you went through all that before. Besides I've stopped now anyway just like I said'.

1. Why do you think that Emma has lied about her smoking?
2. Examine how you feel about Emma's decision to continue smoking while pregnant.
3. Do your feelings reflect a partnership model of care supporting informed choice?
4. Do you think that your approach to Emma's care has encouraged her to feel like a good mother?

From the perspective of women-centered care that is based upon informed choice, women are encouraged to not only be actively involved in their care but also take responsibility for their own wellbeing. Within this policy context responsibility for pregnancy and birth is not exclusively the domain of a midwife or doctor. Instead pregnancy and birth experts provide advice, leaving the pregnant woman faced with the responsibility of having to make up her own mind about her wellbeing. On the face of it informed choice appears to enhance personal freedom and individual development. In practice this policy agenda expects pregnant women to place ever-tighter restrictions on their life styles during pregnancy. Ironically mothers have no choice but to choose, provided that is, that those choices comply with the list of recommendations set out by the midwife.

The moral loading of choice

The moral underpinning of midwifery practice is explicit in midwives' response to choices that they judge threaten the wellbeing of the unborn fetus, such as mothers' choosing to smoke, drink alcohol, take illicit drugs or even eat without censure during pregnancy. In such cases midwives seek to change these behaviours and in extreme cases instigate action that results in babies being removed from their mother's care after birth. For example in Stengel's (2014) study of 13 pregnant women with a drug-taking history, 9 of them feared that their baby would be taken away and in 5 cases this happened. This form of 'policing' does not fit comfortably with midwives preferred role as the mother's trusted adviser. Public health activity here appears to cultivate a relationship of mutual distrust, a far cry from a partnership model of women-centered care. Within such a public health policy context it is not surprising that the women involved in Stengel's study sought to control information about their lives to reduce midwives' surveillance and the risk of the loss of their baby.

While some women resist the medical risk discourse of pregnancy and associated moral judgements of their behaviour, most accept and internalise it. Choice of place of birth is a graphic example of this. Despite 20 years of health policy that encourages choice in where to birth, a policy focus that has culminated in the National Institute for Health and Care Excellence (NICE, 2014) intrapartum guidelines where home birth is recognised as being the safest place to have a baby, the majority of women continue to choose to give birth within the medicalised environment of an acute care setting. Home birth rates in England for example have remained virtually static at 2.5 per cent. By way of explanation for the resilience of the medical risk discourse that surrounds birth in our country, Coxon and her colleagues (2014) draw on empirical narrative research with pregnant women in England to examine the ways in which women's choices about where to give birth were shaped by what they considered safe and normal:

> When women planned hospital birth, they often conceptualised birth as medically risky, and did not raise concerns about overuse of birth interventions; instead, these were considered an essential form of rescue from the uncertainties of birth. Those who planned birth in alternative settings also emphasised their intention, and obligation, to seek medical care if necessary.
>
> (Coxon et al., 2014, p. 51)

Similarly when women reflected on their lifestyle choices during pregnancy they also tended to accept the medical risk discourse. Hammer and Inglin (2014) examined the ways in which pregnancy affected 50 white well-educated Swiss women's smoking and drinking and perception of risk. While all the women in the study tended to reduce or stop these behaviours and see them as risky they differentiated the risks:

> The pregnant women in our study saw smoking during pregnancy as a risk-taking behaviour and a failure to act in the best interest of the foetus. In contrast, under certain conditions, they saw moderate drinking of alcohol during pregnancy as acceptable and responsible behaviour.
>
> (Hammer and Inglin, 2014, p. 22)

Pregnant women's internalisation of the dominant medical discourse to risk can be seen as a form of self-policing, where women are encouraged to not only be actively involved in their care but also take responsibility for their own wellbeing, a form of subordination through the act of self-surveillance. By drawing from broad appeal notions of self-help, collaboration, empowerment and participation and so on, contemporary health policy has achieved both public endorsement and cooperation (Petersen and Lupton, 1996). Thus 'Personal autonomy ... is not antithetical to political power, but rather is part of its exercise since power operates most effectively when subjects actively participate in the process of governance' (Petersen and Lupton, 1996, p. 11).

According to this critique, the policy priorities of informed choice and women-centered care do not represent a shift away from the medical, technocratic discourse of childbirth. On the contrary, this policy agenda represents a voluntary, even self-congratulatory move towards a more subtle but none the less more intense medicalisation. Through self-scrutiny pregnant women actively participate in the medicalised regulation of their own bodies and lifestyles. Box 9.2 highlights some key points related to women's choice in pregnancy and childbirth.

Box 9.2　Key points for women's choice in pregnancy and childbirth

- The women's rhetoric of choice is central to current social policy and finds expression in concepts such as self-help and collaboration
- Women are free to choose as long as their choice is considered to be safe and responsible for the fetus and therefore fits with expert risk assessments
- Client autonomy in the form of woman-centered care, operates as a form of self-discipline
- Midwives give information and choice but maintain surveillance through the clinical gaze to ensure the safety of the pregnant woman and her baby

---

Risk and maternity health policy

Central to contemporary maternity health policy is the issue of risk and risk management. In the next part of this chapter we examine this issue of risk, in particular the technologies of risk management within the maternity care services, to ascertain what insight this can offer in the quest for understanding maternity care provision in the UK.

Health policy experts concur that the influence of risk in healthcare and health policy has expanded to unprecedented levels in the past 20 or so years. Nowhere is this hypersensitivity to risk and interest in risk management more apparent than in maternity care, which is considered to be one of the highest risk areas of care in the NHS (NHS Litigation Authority, 2012). With the introduction of National Service Framework policy guidelines, audit through the Care Quality Commission, establishment of the Litigation Authority with its Clinical Negligence Scheme for Trusts (CNST) and best practice standards of NICE, the maternity services have become firmly entrenched within clinical governance.

The policy reforms of the 1990s involved replacing clinical autonomy, practitioner's use of their clinical judgement based on their clinical knowledge and experience, with collectively agreed clinical guidelines, based on the systematic review of available evidence. Within this policy context clinical decision making follows set algorithmic rules where care pathways are predetermined. Through the institutional standardisation of clinical practice, professional discretion is confined to what has been termed 'scientific-bureaucratic knowledge' (Harrison and Doswell, 2002) or encoded knowledge (Lam, 2000).

An example of how such algorithmic rules circumscribe clinical decision making can be seen in the current management of pregnancies that run beyond 40 weeks of gestation. Whereas historically midwives viewed pregnancy length as something that was individual to the woman, allowing for differentiation from one pregnancy to the other, all practitioners now expect pregnancy to be terminated within a set timeframe. That timeframe is set out in the NICE guidelines, which are reduced down to a clinical decision-making pathway.

Application to practice

We recommend that you consider this practice exercise before reading the rest of the chapter to enhance your understanding. Read the scenario below and consider the numbered points listed at the bottom of this box.

Sandra is expecting her second baby following a straightforward pregnancy. Sandra's previous labour was induced for post term. Sandra has already disclosed to you, her midwife, that she finds the memories of her first labour traumatic and that she believes that this is because she was induced. Sandra comes to see you at 40 weeks gestation and you offer her a stretch and sweep and to refer her to obstetric care for post term.

At this point Sandra breaks down in tears and refuses to accept either of your suggestions. You point out to her that this is the recommended pathway for this point in her pregnancy and she leaves the clinic without making any further appointments to see you.

1. Why do you think that Sandra has chosen to reject your advice?
2. Why did you as the midwife feel obliged to refer Sandra to a service that she was likely to find distressing?
3. What would Sandra's options be now?
4. Does Sandra have the right to refuse this referral even if it puts her unborn child's life at risk?
5. Do your feelings reflect a partnership model of care supporting informed choice?
6. Do you think that your approach to Sandra's care has encouraged her to feel like a good mother?

Clinical governance gave primacy to publically available and verifiable knowledge over more personal types of knowledge such as intuition or custom and practice. While clinical governance reduces the autonomy of individual practitioners, it increased the collective power of the medical profession over childbirth. Acceptable ways of managing birth must now be supported by evidence-based practice where knowledge is collected using predominantly the medical gold standard of randomised controlled trials or, even better, a systematic review of a range of random controlled trials.

The Department of Health led the process of systematically coding knowledge. The first set of guidelines known as National Service Frameworks were for cancer treatment and the process was led by the English and Welsh chief medical officers (Sir Kenneth Calman and Dame Deidre Hine). Subsequently clinical directors (so-called clinical tsars) have played a key role in developing and ensuring the implementation of guidelines. At the same time, the government established a new 'arms-length' body, independent but government funded, to systematically review evidence about specific treatment, initially known as the National Institute for Clinical Excellence.

To ensure the public could trust the system as dependable and that 'bad apples' (such as Harold Shipman) did not escape detection for long, the reforms specified that both the risks and outcomes of clinical decision making should be systematically reviewed. At local level this involved the establishment of clinical governance committees to systematically monitor clinical outcomes and to identify risks and take action to mitigate them. This involved investigating not only adverse events, that is an event in which patients were harmed, but also 'near misses', events in which things went wrong and patients could have been harmed. This local system was overseen by a new body, the Commission for Health Improvement (now the Care Quality Commission) whose role was to investigate any identified unusual patterns of clinical outcomes where there was public concern about the performance of practitioners or hospitals. Although midwives might like to think of themselves as autonomous practitioners delivering individualised care to women and their families, within the contemporary policy context they become agents of clinical governance responsible for delivering standardised care that excludes professional discretion or creative thinking.

The shift from uncertainty to risk

Clinical governance health policy, where the standardisation of decision making is valued over and above professional discretion, has significantly changed the way birth can be managed. Whereas once the potential hazards that always come with childbirth might be thought of in terms of the inevitable uncertainties inherent in the process of reproduction, these hazards have now been recast. The hazards of childbirth can no longer be thought of as chance misfortunes, instead they are understood in terms of risk. This means that poor outcomes tend to be investigated through the risk management system. Within this working environment there is no place for chance, uncertainty or accidents, instead there are only risks that need to be anticipated, planned for and mitigated. Every parent expects a perfect baby and if this does not happen then it is assumed that someone is culpable and should be held to account.

Application to practice

We recommend that you consider this practice exercise before reading the rest of the chapter to enhance your understanding. Read the scenario below and consider the numbered points listed at the bottom of this box.

Laura is birthing her baby at home in a birthing pool. She is progressing well and you judge by her behavior that she has reached full dilatation. As Laura begins to push spontaneously her membranes rupture. You notice that there is thick meconium staining of the liquor.

You ring for an ambulance and advise Laura to leave the pool. On auscultation you observe a fetal heart rate below 110 bpm. When the ambulance arrives the heart rate remains at around 90 bpm. You attend Laura in the ambulance listening to the fetal heart at regular intervals. The baby is delivered by emergency cesarean section but fails to respond to resuscitation. Postmortem results record cause of death as unknown.

1.   Examine how you feel about this scenario.
2.   Are you wondering about cause of this stillbirth? Could it be the place of birth? Or perhaps the use of water during second stage of labour?
3.   Did you find yourself looking for evidence of poor midwifery care?
4.   Does there have to be a cause? If so why?

The distinction between uncertainty and risk is an important one on two counts. First, uncertainty denotes a future that cannot be predicted, an unknown. Second and by contrast, thinking in terms of risk is a process of mitigating those unknowns, minimising the unpredictability of the future in an attempt to improve outcome. Risk implies activities of security (Giddens, 1991). Or put another way, risk thinking is all about 'colonising the future' (Giddens, 1991, p. 133).

Once birth was reconceptualised in terms of risk, technologies of risk management must be employed. In this context, childbirth has to be managed through a standardisation of care through strict obstetric observation and intervention. Importantly there is no room for accidents in the imagined future dominated by risk. Furthermore, individuals, midwives and obstetricians (as well as the mothers themselves), must be held accountable for any failures in birth and the battery of technologies used to manage birth.

Ironically the shift from uncertainty towards risk in the conceptualisation of childbirth has been accompanied by a statistical decrease in the probability of harms associated with reproduction. The current hypersensitivity to the risk in the maternity services has developed in conjunction with an ever-increasing level of safety. As Cartwright and Thomas point out: 'Danger has always attended childbirth . . . Danger was transformed into biomedically constructed and sanctioned notions of risk. This was more than a semantic shift: Dangers implies a fatalistic outlook on birth, risk implies an activist stance' (Cartwright and Thomas, 2001, p. 218).

Due to the risk-centered policy climate in which contemporary maternity services are delivered 'It is the case that debates about childbirth will most likely continue to pivot around the notion of risk despite the low rates of mortality and morbidity relative to pre-war figures in advanced Western economies' (Lane, 1995, p. 56).

As undesirable outcomes have become less likely, preoccupations with these unlikely outcomes has intensified. Furthermore, this intensification shapes how midwives can practice and imagine the manner in which women give birth. The shift from uncertainty to risk apportions a sense of responsibility, accountability and ultimately blame for those involved in managing risk.

The role of the state in the provision of healthcare expanded in the twentieth century. It has created a large-scale system of surveillance that seeks to ensure that clinician's decisions are structured by nationally agreed protocols and guidelines. Within this structured working environment routine midwifery care operates to strengthen the medicalisation of childbirth.

Conclusion

In this chapter we have examined the impact of UK social policy on the delivery of midwifery care. Through the analysis of the policy reforms it has been possible to see and critique how social policy has helped shape midwifery practice over the past hundred years and more. Through this chapter we have encouraged readers to critically evaluate and reflect upon contemporary maternity services in this country.

While most midwives would like to see themselves as autonomous practitioners who enable the women in their care to have safe births, midwifery practice is in fact shaped by the exercises of state power and public policy. Within the current policy climate preoccupations with clinical governance and risk dominate, meaning that routine midwifery care operates to strengthen the standardisation of childbirth through the strict implementation of risk management. In this chapter is has been possible to show how even the midwifery commitments to women-centered care and informed choice operate as mechanisms of subordination. Power is exercised most effectively when subjects actively participate in the process of governance and compliance and midwives are active agents in the expression of this power.

The influence of risk in health and health policy is ubiquitous and it appears that risk has replaced uncertainty. The aim of risk management is to control uncertainties in the future. Risk connotes risk management technologies, accountability, responsibility and blame. To be a midwife within this policy context is to be a risk manager where midwifery practice might be defined as a process of ensuring that pregnant women both undergo constant medical surveillance and scrutiny and at the same time, conform to the accepted understanding of what it is to be a good mother.

References

Adams, J. (2003) *In Defence of Bad Luck. A society which can't accept that accidents happen is destined to be governed by a stifling culture of blame.* Online at: http://www.spiked-online.com/Articles/00000006E02C.htm

Alaszewski, A. (2001) *Health: Managing the risk paradox: Insights from social science.* University of Kent at Canterbury

Alaszewski, A. (2006) 'Health and risk', in P. Taylor-Gooby and J. Zinn (eds) *Risk in the Social Sciences*, Oxford University Press, Oxford, pp. 160–179

Alaszewski, A. (2007) Risk, uncertainty and knowledge. *Health, Risk & Society* 9 (1) pp. 1–10

Alaszewski, A. and Brown, P. (2012) *Making Health Policy: A Critical Introduction*, Polity Press, Cambridge

Annandale, E. and Clark, J. (1996) What is gender? Feminist theory and the sociology of human reproduction, *Sociology of Health & Illness* 18 (1) pp. 17–44

Cartwright, E. and Thomas, J. (2001) Constructing risk, in R. Devries, C. Benoit, E. van Teijlingen and S. Wrede (eds) *Birth by Design. Pregnancy, Maternity Care and Midwifery in North America and Europe*. Routledge, New York, p. 218

Coxon, K., Sandal, J. and Fulop N.J. (2014) To what extent are women free to choose where to give birth? How discourses of risk, blame and responsibility influence birth place decisions, *Health, Risk & Society* 16 (1) pp. 51–67

Department of Health (2007) *Maternity Matters: Choice, access and continuity of care in a safe service*, HMSO, London

Dietsch, E. and Mulimbalimba-Masururu, L. (2011) The experience of being a traditional midwife: living and working in relationship with women, *Journal of Midwifery and Womens Health* 57 (2) pp. 161–166

Gabe, J. (ed.) (1995) *Medicine, Health, and Risk: Sociological approaches*. Blackwell, Oxford and Cambridge, MA

Giddens, A. (ed.) (1991) *Modernity and Self-identity: Self and society in the late modern age*. Polity, Cambridge

Giddens, A. (1998) *The Third Way: Renewal of Social Democracy*. Polity, Cambridge

Green, J. (1999) From accidents to risk: Public health and preventable injury, *Health, Risk & Society* 1 (1) pp. 25–39

Hammer, R. and Inglin, S. (2014) 'I don't think it's risky, but . . .': Pregnant women's risk perceptions of maternal drinking and smoking, *Health, Risk & Society* 16 (1) pp. 22–35

Harrison, S. and Dowsell, G. (2002) Autonomy and bureaucratic accountability in primary care: What English general practitioners say, *Sociology of Health and Illness* 24, pp. 208–226

Harrison, S. and Wood, B. (2000) Scientific-bureaucratic medicine and UK Health Policy, *Review of Policy Research* 17 (4) pp. 25–42

Heyman, B., Shaw, M., Alaszewski, A. and Titterton, M. (eds) (2010) *Risk, Safety, and Clinical Practice Health care through the Lens of Risk*. 1st edition. Oxford University Press, Oxford

Hill, M. (2013) *The Public Policy Process*. Sixth Edition. Routledge, Abingdon, Oxfordshire

Howlett, M., Ramesh, M. and Perl, A. (eds) (1995) *Studying Public Policy: Policy cycles and policy subsystems*. Cambridge University Press, Cambridge

Katz Rothman, B. (2014) Pregnancy, birth and risk: An introduction, *Health, Risk & Society* 16 (1) pp. 1–6

Kirkham, M. (2009) In fear of difference, *Midwifery Matters* 123 pp. 7–9

Lam, A. (2000) Tacit knowledge, organisational learning and societal institutions: an integrated framework, *Organization Studies* 21 (3) pp. 487–513

Lane, K. (1995) The medical model of the body as a site of risk: a case study of childbirth, in J. Gabe (ed.) *Medicine, Health and Risk: Sociological Approaches*. Blackwell Publishers, Oxford, pp. 53–72

Lupton, D. (1999) Risk and the onology of pregnancy embodiment, in D. Lupton (ed.) *Risk and Sociocultural Theory: New Directions and Perspectives*, Cambridge University Press, Cambridge, pp. 59–85

Marshall, H. and Woollett, A. (2000) Fit to reproduce? The regulative role of pregnancy texts. *Feminism & Psychology* 10 pp. 351–366

NHS Litigation Authority (2012) *Ten Years of Maternity Claims: An Analysis of NHS Litigation Authority Data*, NHS, London

NICE (National Institute for Health and Care Excellence) (2014) *Intrapartum Care: Care of healthy women and their babies during childbirth*. National Institute for Health and Care Excellence, London

Petersen, A. and Lupton, D. (eds) (1996) *The New Public Health: Health and Self in the Age of Risk*. Allen & Unwin, St Leonards

Scamell, M. (2011) The swan effect in midwifery talk and practice: A tension between normality and the language of risk, *Sociology of Health & Illness* 10 (33) pp. 987–1001

Skinner, J. (2003) The midwife in the 'risk' society, *New Zealand College of Midwives Journal* 28 pp. 4–7

Stengel, C. (2014) The risk of being 'too honest': Drug use, stigma and pregnancy, *Health, Risk & Society* 16 (1) pp. 36–50

Walsh, D. (2006) Risk and normality in maternity care: Revisioning risk for normal childbirth, in A. Symon (ed.) *Risk and Choice in Maternity Care*. Ist edition. Churchill Livingstone Elsevier, Edinburgh, pp. 89–99

10 The woman with a disability

Maxine Wallis-Redworth

Aim

This chapter aims to explore the concept of disability by examining some of the perceptions and definitions of disability. It will then move onto look at the relationship of disability and childbearing, highlighting the demographics of those women who embark on childbearing and identifying the experiences of women with a disability. Lastly it will examine how midwives need to consider the woman's unique needs in order to deliver care. This chapter should encourage the reader to reflect upon their experience to date, their current practice and identify possibilities for future practice development, both at a personal and organisational level.

Learning outcomes

By the end of this chapter the reader will be able to:

1. Understand the concept of disability
2. Understand different perceptions of disability
3. Appreciate the experiences of women with disabilities related to childbearing
4. Identify barriers that may impact on delivery of the most appropriate care for women with disabilities
5. Appreciate the guidance available to midwives to provide appropriate care for women with disabilities
6. Reflect on their personal knowledge, skills and attitudes towards women with disabilities

---

Introduction: Defining disability

The road travelled to a twenty-first century understanding of disability has been informed by an evolving societal attitude towards people with disabilities, from a position of non-acknowledgement and isolation to one of greater understanding, acceptance and integration within society.

Historically in Western societies the concept of disability has been viewed negatively as illustrated by words such as 'cripple', 'sufferer' and 'mental handicap'. People with a disability were viewed both as unfortunate because they were dependent on others for their medical and social care, and dysfunctional in terms of societal contribution (Barnes and Mercer, 2003). Thus the correlation between disability and dependence was established by society.

Disability was medicalised perhaps as a consequence of the failure to create a cure and thus, in the absence of a cure, the only option was ongoing medical management. This in itself created dependence for care. Traditionally the concepts of disability and dependence were merged without consideration of the consequences. Independence for people with disabilities was regarded in a more restricted manner, being viewed as their ability to perform tasks of daily living without help, or the extent to which they could participate in day-to-day activities.

Disabled People's International (1982) championed the liberation of the concepts of disability and impairment. An impairment relates to complete or partial loss of physical, mental or sensory function beyond the short-term, while disability was linked to loss or limitation of opportunities to participate in everyday life within a community due to physical and social barriers.

The Disability Discrimination Act (1995) brought a legal definition of disability by defining disability as '... a physical or mental impairment which has a substantial and long-term adverse effect on his ability to carry out normal day-to-day activities'. Again the assumption appears to have been that 'normal' day-to-day activities infer independence. However, Prilleltensky (2003) refers to independence for people with a disability as the capacity to be autonomous in making important life decisions for themselves, rather than independence in a physical activity sense. This philosophy reiterates the emphasis is on the person, not the condition. The Equality Act (2010) reinforced the duty of all members of society to make reasonable adjustments to avoid substantial disadvantage for those members with a disability. This Act also required that where a physical feature could confer substantial disadvantage, then society is required to remove that physical feature, alter it or provide a means to avoid it. This gives the flexibility to come up with a solution that is best for an individual and their circumstances.

The predominant thinking on disability was within the medical model. Further exploration of the concept of disability positioned understanding of disability within a socio-medical model that has both consequence and significance (Bury, 1997). Bury (1997) saw consequence as the impact on a person's everyday roles and relationships, while significance concerns the cultural meanings of specific conditions.

The International Classification of Functioning, Disability and Health of the World Health Organization (WHO) (2001) is an illustration of recognition of the socio-medical model, with a focus on categorising human function according to impairment of bodily structure and/or function, activity limitations and participation restrictions within any area of life. Thus disability emerges when a person has difficulties with all or any of these three areas. As a result of using this as a guiding framework, it is impossible to create a specific definition of disability that can be applied universally.

Its strength is that each person has to be assessed individually to determine where they are on the ability–disability continuum for each component and then making a holistic judgement of overall disabling effect. It helps to promote the idea that not everything about the person is disabling, thus recognising different aspects of ability.

Additionally, the emergence of public health models of care has strengthened the social models of disabling illness, in that public health views disability as just one of many health risks alongside those of poverty and social isolation (Krahn and Campbell, 2011). Thus the integration of the public health philosophy may serve to make disability inclusive rather than exclusive in our society.

Bury's work (1997) also helps to demonstrate that the inclusion of the social model of disability helps practitioners to take a broader view. This social model also recognises that the source of many hindrances/barriers to full and effective participation within society is that same society. However, it is not simply a case that there has been movement from the medical to the social model. Rather, there has been a timely cultural shift of opinion about the value of people with a disability, alongside the recognition of the complexity and diversity within different people's disabling conditions. This has led to an acknowledgement that people with disabilities can experience related and unrelated health and social problems during their lifetime, which may or may not be exacerbated by issues such as societal and individual attitudes and the environments they need to live and work in, and that they may need to adapt.

French and Swain (2008) recognise that the answer to what is disability is a political one with many different stakeholders who have deep-seated interests. These stakeholders range from families, professionals, advocacy and support groups, all of whom have a unique set of values and beliefs that drive their definition of disability. French and Swain (2008) suggest that disability is not simply defined because there is much more at stake including the differing values, professional status, identity, power and control. Perhaps the most important driver is the need to accept that disability is a consequence for the person affected and not their sole defining attribute. Article 1 of the United Nations Convention on the Rights of Persons with Disabilities (2006) identified that disability results from the interaction between persons with long-term impairments and the various barriers that may impede their maximal and successful involvement in society on a par with others. Such barriers have had a powerful influence on the labelling of disability. Barnes and Mercer (2003) identify that the term disabled person is used because it accentuates the ways that social barriers impact life chances. However in this chapter, in keeping with a woman-centred philosophy for midwifery care, the phrase woman/person/people with a disability is used to identify that the woman comes first and the disability second.

It is important to remember that disability is still a 'complex, dynamic, multidimensional and contested' entity (WHO, 2011, p.3). There is a need to recognise that disability takes many forms, such as physical, mental or sensory, overt or hidden and emerges in different ways, for example congenital or acquired. Exact statistics on the number of people with a disabling condition are not known. The WHO (2011) estimates that approximately 16–19 per cent of the world's adult population has a type of disability, with a 9 per cent estimate within the 18–49 year age group. Šumilo et al. (2012) using publically available Millennium Cohort Study data identified that there was a 9.4 per cent prevalence of limiting longstanding illnesses/disability among women giving birth in the United Kingdom (UK) in 2000–2002. Following publication in July 2014 of an opinion from the Court of Justice of the European Union (2014), health and social care practitioners may need to reconsider the causes of disability and thus those people with a disability. The opinion from the advocate general (Court of Justice of the European Union, 2014) saw the origin of disability as irrelevant, thus putting the greater emphasis on the effect of disability. In this opinion, the advocate general (Court of Justice of the European Union, 2014) considered that morbid obesity may be classified as a disability due to the potential for impairment in a person's ability to carry out normal day-to-day activities, such as employment. This is pertinent to midwifery practice as there is acknowledgement that there is a growing percentage of the maternity population who are significantly obese (Heslehurst et al., 2010).

Disability and childbearing

Historically, women with a disability did not engage with childbearing (Morton, et al., 2013). Disability was seen as the barrier to entering into relationships and there was a prevailing attitude that women with a disability were not seen as having the same rights because their disability lessened their rights of personhood (Landsman, 2000). Tepper (2000) identified that the media reinforced the thinking that sexual activity was a privilege for non-disabled people. Sociocultural barriers and attitudes towards sexual activity and sexuality may be as disabling as the impairment itself (Sakellariou, 2006). Kirshbaum and Olkin (2002, p.67) refer to parenting for people with disabilities as 'the last frontier' and one in which they are likely to meet discrimination. Thus stigma attributed to disability extends beyond personhood to parenthood.

For the woman with a disability, Lipson and Rogers (2000) identify three main factors that form an individual woman's experience of childbearing: her specific disability; her resources; and her view of pregnancy and birth. Any other woman's experience is likely to be shaped by issues such as their view of childbearing, their support network and their encounters with other women and the health and social care professionals. Therefore, the one factor that differentiates the woman with a disability from any other childbearing woman is the presence of her specific disability. Thus for the professional it is important to remember that she is a woman who is pregnant and who also has a disability. The nature of her disabling condition may or may not have a significant impact on how her pregnancy progresses, the care she requires and the outcomes for herself and her baby.

A study by Nosek et al (2001) illustrates that there is still a significant gap in the childbearing rate between women with no identifiable disability (51 per cent) and those women with a disability (38 per cent). There are a number of reasons for such a finding. Both women with and without a disability may choose not to embark on childbearing for a variety of personal reasons; equally, the attitudinal response within society of disbelief that the woman with a disability would want to or could have a family may mitigate against the possibility of childbearing. This may be due to the belief that pregnancy complications are more likely and/or an opinion of how successful the woman may be in the mothering role.

This may be an indicator that views held by many people about disability are shaped by stereotypes rather than exact knowledge or personal experience and thus such stereotyping is capable of creating unrealistic and extreme positive or negative views (Lawson, 2001). Equally, Lipson and Rogers study (2000) identified that the initial negativity by family and friends is due to the concern and worry about the impact of the pregnancy on the woman and her health; nevertheless, this can change in later pregnancy to become a positive stance, possibly as the family see that the negative impact does not occur or is not as serious as anticipated. A more recent study by Walsh-Gallagher et al. (2012) elicited positive and congratulatory family attitudes, and this appears to confirm the views of McKay-Moffat and Cunningham (2006) that family attitudes are changing, with more women with a disability embarking on motherhood without a negative or hostile reaction.

Šumilo et al.'s secondary data analysis (2012) explored the characteristics of the women with and without disability. While they found no significant difference in age or ethnicity, they found women with disabilities were more likely to live in poverty and receive benefits, have lower educational attainments and not have planned their pregnancy. Women with disabilities were more likely not to be in a supportive relationship (Redshaw et al., 2013), but if they had a partner, then they were more likely to be subject to domestic violence (Šumilo et al., 2012).

Trigger

Does your maternity unit have a resource file of disability advocacy groups/organisations that will help plan care for a woman with a disability? If not, how would you go about creating one?

Experiences of women

Women with disabilities can be assumed to be no different to other pregnant women in how they embark on a journey to attain their mothering role and what their desires are for their unborn child. When any prospective parent is asked if they are hoping for a boy or girl, the answer is usually 'I don't mind, as long as the baby is healthy'. This frames the response in terms of health of the baby rather than sex, helping to reiterate the societal desire for ability rather than disability. This is not surprising given that health is viewed 'as a priceless possession (and) . . . good health is the ultimate commodity' (Tighe, 2001, p. 511).

Research has been undertaken into the views of women with a disability in relation to pregnancy and birth experience and that of parenting. Women with a disability have expressed the same desire as other women, namely normality, along with independence and acceptance as mothers (Thomas, 1997). Mayes et al. (2011) identified that pregnant women with an intellectual disability do assume a protective and nurturing stance towards their unborn baby in working towards attaining identity as a mother and working towards taking on the mantle of motherhood.

Thomas (1997) gave a helpful insight into the views of women with disabilities who were anticipating motherhood, or already engaged on that journey. The women considered they were taking a risk due to either the hereditary nature of their condition or the potential harmful effect of their medication regimen. Women with an obvious physical disability reported that their doctor expressed shock when they told them of the pregnancy and automatically assumed they would want either a termination of pregnancy or antenatal testing for fetal abnormality to ensure they did not create a further problem. The women felt that a lack of precise knowledge about their specific disability was the reason for the response (Prilleltensky, 2003; Smeltzer, 2007; Walsh-Gallagher et al., 2012). However, the offering of a termination of pregnancy is not universal. McKay-Moffat and Cunningham (2006) noted a significant change of practice from that reported in an earlier study (Rotherham, 1989), with none of the women in their study having been offered a termination of pregnancy.

Lack of accurate and helpful information from doctors, nurses and midwives has been a theme women with a disability have reported over the decades. In a more recent study midwives identified they lacked general disability knowledge and awareness, which impacted on the quality of care provision (McKay-Moffat and Cunningham, 2006). Many of the women in Thomas's study (1997) reported receiving conflicting information that did not enable them to make wise choices and that, as a consequence of poor information, they had to live with the guilt of a baby born with impairments. Some women identified that they needed to make compromises in order to promote optimal normality for their unborn baby, and that this could give rise to negative consequences to their long-term maternal health.

Historically not all experiences of working towards motherhood were positive ones. Many of the women were aware that they were engaging with professionals driven by the medical risk model and that their decision to be pregnant or continue with their pregnancy was often perceived as risky by health professionals (Thomas, 1997). This attitude of risk appears to be changing with many women with disabilities not being labelled as high risk on the basis of the disability alone (Smeltzer, 2002). The women in Thomas' study (1997) also expressed a fear of being judged as a mother and the potential consequences of being viewed as an inadequate mother. This fear of judgement was from both professionals and family, with some women identifying interference from families who did not believe they could or would cope. The women felt vulnerable in that they recognised the need for specific help in order to undertake all parenting tasks, but it was not necessarily forthcoming. When help came the women felt it was often unhelpful, as other people took over. However, these women recognised that many health and social care professionals were well intentioned but lacked specific information or skills they needed for successful parenting. The women required good communication as a partner in her care in order to identify where she was on the ability–inability continuum and to promote maximal independence for herself and in caring for her baby.

In a recent study (Walsh-Gallagher et al., 2012) the women identified two major themes – affirmation of motherhood and fear of motherhood. They celebrated conception after being told so often that pregnancy may never occur, and while pregnant they saw that their impending motherhood illustrated their femininity. Giving birth produced a sense of achievement in terms of their role as a woman, wife/partner and mother. This sense of achievement appeared to assist the bonding with their baby and all of these aspects translated into confidence in their new role.

However, such positivity was offset by the reality check that these mothers experienced through the negative reactions of other people. In particular, the women perceived that professional concerns for their wellbeing and that of the baby were often founded on a lack of knowledge. A lack of practical information and support also increased their sense of isolation. This illustrates an unchanging situation from the 1990s when Thomas (1997) undertook her research.

In addition these women worried about the increased surveillance of their mothering; this is an aspect that had been highlighted a decade earlier by Kirshbaum and Olkin (2002) when women with a disability who successfully birthed their babies reported that they had to endure scrutiny as to their suitability to be a 'hands on' mother.

There is wide acknowledgement that women with disabilities can face additional challenges to those without disabilities, albeit dependent on the nature of their disability and the support network they have in place. In a recent study (Mayes et al., 2011) mothers with intellectual disabilities were interviewed in an attempt to explore the development of their mothering identity. None of these mothers expected to raise their child alone due to the nature of their disability – they were realistic in realising that they needed a strong support network around them. These women found that having social support and a specific ally/advocate who acknowledged their pregnancy, supported them and saw them as the pivotal person in their baby's life was essential to help develop their mothering skills.

Therefore for women with disabilities, family and health professionals who constantly challenge or undermine their ability to protect and nurture their unborn child, can negatively impact the woman's journey. The quality of the social support network a pregnant woman is surrounded by is significant in how well she embraces and adapts to her mothering role.

Having identified that many women with disabilities have a less than positive experience with the maternity services, it is crucial that midwives are able to respond to the vision set out in *Midwifery 2020* (Chief Nursing Officers of England, Northern Ireland, Scotland and Wales, 2010) and fulfil the role as the coordinator of care for such women.

How midwives can deliver care for the woman with a disability

Midwifery support for a woman with a disability needs to be based on full acknowledgement of that woman's rights – the right to parent and the associated responsibility to parent (Tarleton and Ward, 2007). Once professionals incorporate this basic philosophy into their approaches a partnership model is attainable. Unfortunately there are too many cases where support when offered, was often reactionary in nature and frequently in response to a crisis rather than being proactive in nature (Tarleton and Ward, 2007). This probably reflects the lack of specific knowledge referred to earlier in the chapter.

If midwives believe that all women accessing the maternity services in the UK matter, and all women need to have an individualised assessment of their history and needs, then there is no need to make a significant alteration to the nature of care women with a disability can expect to receive from midwives. This should not be a challenge in current maternity services given that maternity care should be woman centred and evidence based (Chief Nursing Officers of England, Northern Ireland, Scotland and Wales, 2010). There is much talk of working in partnership with women and in the case of women with a disability then the 'expert midwife' must be prepared to see the 'expert client' as an equal in order to assess, plan, implement and evaluate the care package that fulfils everyone's agenda.

Unfortunately, there is recognition that a number of issues can create additional challenges for women with a disability in accessing maternity services. These include availability of suitable transport, the physical design of buildings and interior layouts, availability of additional equipment to assist in access or care provision, in addition to the variation in staff knowledge and attitudes towards disability (Redshaw et al., 2013). These are also challenges for the midwives, but within the application of the Equality Act (2010), midwives at both managerial and clinical levels need to rise to the challenges and seek and use both strategic and operational measures to eliminate substantial disadvantage to the woman with a disability.

Application to practice

Women with disabilities are experts in their own condition and can define their own normality and need to be significant players in the assessment, planning, implementation and evaluation of their maternity care.

Think about a time you witnessed a consultation between a woman with a disability and a healthcare professional. Was the woman treated as a significant player and an expert in her own condition in this interaction?

For midwives, caring for women with disabilities requires seeing the pregnant client at the centre of a small support team – a team that only the pregnant woman can determine membership of. The pregnant women/mothers in Mayes et al.'s study (2011) chose the members of their support team carefully and at times changed that membership when they realised the potential negative impact of the presence of a particular team member on the future of their child. Midwives thus need to be equally prepared to be flexible and adapt to who constitutes the support team, thus showing respect for the woman and her right to autonomy.

Does your maternity unit have up-to-date information that addresses the care needs of specific disabilities within the antenatal, intrapartum and postnatal areas?

Taking a woman-centred approach should ensure that the unique circumstances of the woman and the unique nature of her disabling condition is central to the holistic assessment, planning and implementation of a personalised care package. The care package has to be planned in a proactive and sensitive manner, at all times seeking to empower rather than disempower or further disable the woman. All care should be underpinned by the six Cs from *Compassion in Practice* (Commissioning Board, Chief Nursing Officer and DH Chief Nursing Adviser, 2012). It is clear from the research identified earlier women with disabilities want care, compassion, competence, communication, courage and commitment from all staff.

Does your local Maternity Services Liaison Committee have a woman with disabilities within the group? If not, how does this group make sure that the needs of this group of women are not overlooked?

In an ideal world, the woman with a disability should be able to discuss her prospective childbearing with her medical team as well as a midwife and obstetrician in order to increase her informed decision making. Preconception care is a key to attaining good health, identifying specific risks and possible ways to reduce such risk (Barrowclough, 2009), more so for women with disabilities as research has identified that a significant proportion of women with a disability did not plan their pregnancies (Šumilo et al., 2012).

Preconception care needs to be a team approach involving professionals such as the woman's general practitioner, the consultant for her disability condition, the obstetrician, midwife, anaesthetist and other allied health and social care professionals such as physiotherapist, occupational therapist, as well as social workers or other key workers. Thierry (2006) asserts that a deep understanding of the condition and a thorough knowledge of disabling conditions combined with a multidisciplinary approach to pregnancy management are essential elements for good pregnancy outcomes. Preconception care needs to utilise a holistic approach using a biopsychosocial framework that identifies both actual and potential issues before, during and after a pregnancy, enabling the woman and her partner to receive realistic information about the chances of success and problems. The Common Assessment framework (Department for Education and Skills, 2006) is a recognised tool that will enable the midwife to make a more holistic assessment and coordinate appropriate care. The social aspects of preconception care should not be marginalised as by assessing and planning to maintain or even improve a woman's social support network can improve the overall quality of her life. Previous research has illustrated that quality of life for people with a disability was enhanced with integral social support, while the absence of social support resulted in a poorer quality of life (Albrecht and Devlieger, 1999).

In regards to antenatal and labour care, Redshaw et al. (2013) identified differences and similarities between women with a disability and those without. While women with a disability did not differ in timing of first contact with a health professional or for their booking appointment, they had more contact antenatally, more ultrasound scans, less choice of place of birth and fewer of the women attended preparation for parenthood classes. For birth outcomes, women with a disability were more likely to have a planned caesarean section, possibly due to the physical limitations of their disability. Specifically more women with a physical disability had met labour ward staff prior to their labours. This was presumably as part of planning their environment and assessing equipment needs/usage. There should be no difference for women with a disability of a mental health origin, as preparation for and familiarity with the environment and staff could be an equally important feature of birth planning. Postnatally women with a disability had longer hospital stays and were less likely to breastfeed.

In attempting to address how to provide care during childbearing to women with a disability care there is a temptation to be prescriptive in order to minimise risk but this does not promote woman-centred/individualised care. If the midwifery care of a woman with a disability is assessed, planned and implemented in the same way as any other woman then a general framework can be used with the awareness that 'one size does not fit all'.

Provision of antenatal care may need to be adapted around the woman's needs if there are environmental access barriers that prevent her from attending a physical venue for care; for example, a woman with a physical disability may require a ramp to access the building and a lift to access rooms above ground floor level. Physical examination may be precluded if there is no height-adjustable examination table or suitable hoist with trained healthcare personnel to assist the woman. It is useful to remember that not all health and social settings in the community are disabled-access friendly buildings.

Intrapartum care needs to be proactively planned and the choice of venues debated to ensure a practical choice is made and the additional equipment needed is available. Such discussions are ideally within the birthing environment as it offers an opportunity for the woman to give the facilities a 'test-run' and identify what adaptations need to be made for her. Generally this puts an emphasis on the woman with physical mobility limitation, but is also crucial for the visually impaired woman in order for her to plan how she can be mobile, or for the woman who is deaf to plan how she can successfully communicate through lip reading if the room was flooded with strong sunlight or during the night when only a lamp lights the room to promote a relaxed ambience.

Postnatally the plan of care should consider what specific disability condition care the woman may require and thus how easy it is to access such care from within the maternity care setting or at home. Knowledge of how the woman manages her daily care needs to be woven in and if she has specific carers then enabling them to provide care within the maternity unit may promote her independence and sense of control. Very specific care needs may necessitate the allocation of a single room to ensure privacy and dignity, as well as enabling her wider support team to be with her outside of the formal visiting hours for the maternity unit. Additionally infant feeding support may require specialist advice and support or even additional time from maternity support workers or breastfeeding peer supporters to enable mother and baby to establish effective infant feeding within individual limitations. Women with a disability initially may require more frequent home visits to ease the transition to motherhood, rather than be expected to attend children's centres.

Whilst standard pregnancy and postnatal information is appropriate for the 'able mother', there is a need to recognise the small but significant number of women with a disability who may use the local maternity services each year.

Within the UK both the Royal College of Midwives (RCM) and the Royal College of Nursing (RCN) have published guidance papers to assist midwives and nurses to provide appropriate care to women with disabilities. The RCM's guidance *Maternity Care for Disabled Women* (2008) identifies recommendations for good practice covering organisational/service delivery and specific midwifery practice in caring for women with disabilities. The RCN guidance (2007, pp. 13–14) *Pregnancy and Disability* contains key points for antenatal care that involve:

> early identification of women with a disability, referral to a specialist midwife with responsibility for disability, using the woman's assessment of her needs and her strengths, discussion with the woman of a comprehensive plan of care to cover care at home and in hospital from pregnancy to the postnatal period, liaison with both the woman and the multidisciplinary team to meet her complex needs, and provision of antenatal/intrapartum care at a location that is mutually suitable e.g., home.

Trigger

Does your maternity unit have a specialist midwife who focuses on the needs of women with a disability?

Despite this guidance, while some areas of the UK have a disability specialist midwife in place to support both women and other midwives, there are still serious gaps in the provision of appropriate and sensitive individualised maternity care for women with disabilities. Based on studies over the last 15 years, there appears to be a need to address specific information needs relating to labour and postnatal care (Lipson and Rogers, 2000; Walsh-Gallagher et al., 2012). In 2013 Walsh-Gallagher et al. identified a continuing lack of knowledge about specific disabilities, lack of communication, lack of support and non-individualised care. More recently Malouf et al. (2014) concurred in their review that healthcare providers are often unfamiliar with the needs of women with disability. They also identified that there is a shortage of good evidence of appropriate approaches to support the care of women with disabilities during childbearing due to the limited number of studies that focus on care delivery to a significant cohort of women with a disability.

Application to practice

While there are good practice examples emerging across the UK, further improvements in the quality of care for women with disabilities can and must be made. How would you achieve this in your workplace?

Conclusion

Women with a disability have the same desires as their childbearing sisters without disabilities – to have a positive experience of pregnancy, labour and birth, and motherhood. Women with a disability have their own normality and are realistic about what they can achieve but also have aspirations. They expect to receive supportive midwifery care that provides acceptance of their condition, acknowledgement of their personal expertise of their disabling condition and a desire to work as a part of their team to achieve a healthy outcome. These women want to be cared for by knowledgeable practitioners who provide accurate information and flexible care. Midwives need to work within a multidisciplinary team to provide the most appropriate care for these women.

While the numbers of women with disabling conditions accessing a maternity unit remain small, nationally the numbers will continue to rise. There is a need to share examples of successful practice in order to positively impact other women in other localities.

References

Albrecht, G.L. and Devlieger, P.J., 1999. The disability paradox: high quality of life against all odds. *Social Science and Medicine*. 48(8), pp.977–988.

Barnes, C. and Mercer, G., 2003. *Disability*. Malden, MA: Polity Press.

Barrowclough, D., 2009. Preparing for pregnancy. In. D. Fraser and M.A. Cooper eds. *Myles textbook for midwives, 15th edn*. Edinburgh: Churchill Livingstone Elsevier.

Bury, M., 1997. *Health and Illness in a Changing Society*. London: Routledge.

Chief Nursing Officers of England, Northern Ireland, Scotland and Wales. 2010. *Midwifery 2020*. London: Department of Health.

Commissioning Board, Chief Nursing Officer and DH Chief Nursing Adviser, 2012. *Compassion in Practice. Nursing, Midwifery and Care Staff Our Vision and strategy*. Leeds: Department of Health.

Court of Justice of the European Union, 2014. Advocate General's Opinion in Case C-354/13. FOA, acting on behalf of Karsten Kaltoft v Kommunernes Landsforening (KL), acting on behalf of the Municipality of Billund. Press release 112/14. Luxembourg. Online at: http://curia.europa.eu/jcms/jcms/Jo2_16799/?annee=2014

Department for Education and Skills, 2006. *Working Together to Safeguard Children.* London: HMSO.

Disabled People's International, 1982. *Proceedings of the First World Congress.* Singapore: Disabled People's International.

French, S. and Swain, J., 2008. *Understanding Disability: Guide for health professionals.* Edinburgh: Churchill Livingstone Elsevier.

Heslehurst, N., Rankin, J., Wilkinson, J.R. and Summerbell, C.D., 2010. A nationally representative study of maternal obesity in England, UK: trends in incidence and demographic inequalities in 619,323 births, 1989–2007. *International Journal of Obesity,* 34(3), pp.420–428.

Kirshbaum, M. and Olkin, R., 2002. Parents with physical, systemic, or visual disabilities. *Sexuality and Disability,* 20(1), pp. 65–80.

Krahn, G. and Campbell, V.A., 2011. Evolving views of disability and public health: The roles of advocacy and public health. *Disability and Health Journal,* 4(1), pp.12–18.

Landsman, G.H., 2000. 'Real motherhood,' class, and children with disabilities. In H. Ragone and F.W. Twine, eds, *Ideologies and Technologies of Motherhood: Race, class, sexuality, nationalism.* London: Routledge.

Lawson, K.L., 2001. Contemplating selective reproduction: the subjective appraisal of parenting a child with a disability. *Journal of Reproductive and Infant Psychology,* 19(1), pp.73–82.

Lipson, J.G. and Rogers, J.G., 2000. Pregnancy, birth, and disability: Women's health care experiences. *Health Care for Women International,* 21(1), pp.11–26.

McKay-Moffat, S. and Cunningham, C., 2006. Services for women with disabilities: mothers' and midwives' experiences. *British Journal of Midwifery,* 14(8), pp.472–477.

Malouf, R., Redshaw, M., Kurinczuk, J. and Gray, R., 2014. Systematic review of health care interventions to improve outcomes for women with disability and their family during pregnancy, birth and postnatal period. *BMC Pregnancy and Childbirth,* 14, p.58.

Mayes, R., Llewellyn, G. and McConnell, D., 2011. 'That's who I chose to be': The mother identity for women with intellectual disabilities. *Women's Studies International Forum,* 34(2), pp.112–120.

Morton, C., Le, J.T., Shahbandar, L., Hammond, C., Murphy, E. and Kirschner, K.L., 2013. Pregnancy outcomes of women with physical disabilities: A matched cohort study. *Physical Medicine and Rehabilitation,* 5(2), pp.90–98.

Nosek, M.A., Howland, B.A., Rinalta, D.H., Young, M.E. and Chanpong, M.S., 2001. National study of women with physical disabilities: final report. *Sexuality and Disability,* 19(1), pp.5–39.

Prilleltensky, O., 2003. A ramp to motherhood: the experiences of mothers with physical disabilities. *Sexuality and Disability,* 21(1), pp.21–47.

RCM (Royal College of Midwives), 2008. *Maternity Care for Disabled Women.* London: RCM.

RCN (Royal College of Nursing), 2007. *Pregnancy and Disability. RCN guidance for midwives and nurses.* London: RCN.

Redshaw, M., Malouf, R., Gao, H. and Gray, R., 2013. Women with disability: the experience of maternity care during pregnancy, labour and birth and the postnatal period. *BMC Pregnancy and Childbirth,* 13, p.174.

Rotherham, J. 1989. Care of the disabled woman during pregnancy. *Nursing Standard,* 4(10), pp.36–39.

Sakellariou, D., 2006. If not the disability, then what? Barriers to reclaiming sexuality following spinal cord injury. *Sexuality and Disability*, 24(2), pp.101–111.

Smeltzer, S.C., 2007. Pregnancy in women with physical disabilities. *Journal of Obstetric, Gynecologic and Neonatal Nursing*, 36 (1), pp.88–96.

Šumilo, D., Kurinczuk, J., Redshaw, M. and Gray, R., 2012. Prevalence and impact of disability in women who had recently given birth in the UK. *BMC Pregnancy and Childbirth*, 12, p.31.

Tarleton, B. and Ward, L., 2007. 'Parenting with support': The views and experiences of parents with intellectual disabilities. *Journal of Policy and Practice in Intellectual Disabilities*, 4(3), pp.194–202.

Tepper, M., 2000. Sexuality and disability: the missing discourse of pleasure. *Sexuality and Disability*, 18(4), pp.283–290.

Thierry, J., 2006. The importance of preconception care for women with disabilities. *Maternal Child Health Journal*, 10(5) Supplement, pp.S175–S176.

Thomas, C., 1997. The baby and the bath water: disabled women and motherhood in social context. *Sociology of Health & Illness*, 19(5), pp.622–643.

Tighe, C.A., 2001. 'Working at disability': a qualitative study of the meaning of health and disability for women with physical impairments. *Disability & Society*, 16(4), pp.511–529.

United Nations, 2006. *The United Nations Convention on the Rights of Persons with Disabilities*. New York: United Nations.

Walsh-Gallagher, D., Sinclair, M. and McConkey, R., 2012. The ambiguity of disabled women's experiences of pregnancy, childbirth and motherhood: a phenomenological understanding. *Midwifery*, 28(2), pp.156–162.

Walsh-Gallagher, D., McConkey, R., Sinclair, M. and Clarke, R., 2013. Normalising birth for women with a disability: the challenges facing practitioners. *Midwifery*, 29(4), pp.294–299.

World Health Organization, 2001. *The International Classification of Functioning, Disability and Health*. Geneva: WHO.

World Health Organization, 2011. *World Report on Disability*. Geneva: WHO Press.

11 Sexuality and midwifery

Susan Walker and Mary Stewart

Aim

This chapter unravels what sexuality is and why it is relevant to the practice of midwifery today. It also uses some specific case studies to help the reader think through the relevance of sexuality in midwifery.

Learning outcomes

By the end of this chapter the reader will be able to:

- Think about sexuality in a variety of frameworks
- Understand how these frameworks influence one another and how they impact upon midwifery practice
- Reflect on what good professional care might mean in the context of caring for a lesbian couple
- Reflect upon how stigma and discrimination can be tackled in a midwifery setting
- Reflect upon the impact of sexuality in a midwifery setting

---

Introduction

Trigger

Think about what a 'working definition' of sexuality might be. If you were explaining it to an alien visitor for whom it was an unknown concept, what would you say?

Sexuality is a quality of human beings that goes beyond activity or behaviour involving the genital organs. Here are some suggestions. Sexuality is:

- Related to reproduction (but only sometimes)
- Related to gender (but not straightforwardly e.g. people are not only attracted to the 'opposite sex')
- Important to intimate, loving relationships (but not all kinds e.g. not between parents and children)
- Capable of providing intense physical pleasure and wellbeing (but not to everyone and not all the time)
- An intrinsic part of human identity and self-experience (to a greater or lesser extent)

Within sexuality are a number of different terms that are sometimes confused. These aspects of sexuality are:

- Gender
- Gender identity
- Sexual acts
- Sexual practice
- Sexual orientation

Gender

Gender refers to whether a person is viewed as female or male and is usually based on biological sex markers (e.g. clitoris or penis, vagina or scrotum). The term is preferable to 'sex' because it includes the social aspects of gender. Girls wearing pink and teenage boys crying less easily than teenage girls are not biological phenomena but are highly gendered social realities. In most societies people are gendered either female or male but in some societies the picture is more complex. Occasionally biological sex is not straightforward and babies are born with a mixture of female and male sexual markers e.g. hermaphrodites, but most people are forced to live as one gender or the other.

Gender identity

Gender identity is connected to gender, and refers to the gender the person feels her or himself to be. Gender identity is usually established very early in life, and there is debate over whether it is primarily a biological or a social phenomenon. If a person's gender identity differs from her or his biological sex, this can cause great distress. Some people whose gender identity differs from their biological sexual identity will seek to live as the gender they feel themselves to be. They are referred to as transgendered people or transsexual people, if the discrepancy becomes known or is disclosed. 'Trans' people may or may not self-identify as such. Accessing health services can be very problematic for 'trans' people, and may require self-disclosure if the medical procedure or treatment necessitate revealing the disjuncture between lived gender and biological sex. For example some 'trans' men still require a cervical smear.

Sexual acts

Sexual acts are the behaviours that people engage in to achieve sexual pleasure and satisfaction. Within the field of health these are most usually thought of as acts involving penile-vaginal intercourse ending in orgasm, but this is because health professionals most often focus upon the reproductive aspect of sexuality. Sexual acts can also involve other parts of the body (kissing, oral sex, hand-genital contact) and may involve one (masturbation), two or, sometimes, more than two people. Sometimes the giving of flowers, holding hands, dancing, hugging, sharing a strand of spaghetti and many other behaviours can be thought of as 'sexual' depending on the context. The wide range and contextual nature of what may be thought of as sexual means that sexuality is dispersed and ubiquitous. It also means that what is thought of as sexual by one person may not be interpreted as such by another. This can sometimes cause misunderstanding and distress.

Sexual practice

Sexual practice is related to sexual acts in that it refers to the sexual acts that a person commonly performs. Some sexual practices may have implications for sexual health e.g. anal, oral or vaginal intercourse, use of sex toys, use of condoms, monogamy or non-monogamy. Many sexual practices may have few health implications but can cause problems in terms of moral judgement, stigma or discrimination e.g. sadomasochism, role play, masturbation or use of pornography.

Sexual orientation

Sexual orientation is usually taken to refer to the gender of the person to whom one is attracted, in relation to one's own gender. At its most basic sexual orientation is heterosexual if a person is attracted to a person of a different (Greek = *hetero*) gender, and homosexual if a person is attracted to a person of the same (Greek = *homo*) gender. It is important to remember that sexual orientation is much more nuanced than this, in that a person can have both heterosexual and homosexual attractions, that sexual orientation can vary over a lifetime, and that sexual orientation can form the basis of self-identity and peer group identity, and impacts on many aspects of life beyond the field of sexual behaviour. The use of the word 'homosexual' is rather old fashioned, except in a purely descriptive sense, and the labels of lesbian, gay, 'queer', 'bi', 'LBGT' and so on are more usual, more usually self-applied and perhaps less medicalising.

It is also important to realise that a person's primary sexual orientation may not be reflected in the sexual behaviour that they engage in, or are permitted to engage in. In other words people with heterosexual orientation may engage in sexual behaviour with members of the same gender for a variety of reasons, and people with homosexual orientation may engage mostly or exclusively in heterosexual behaviour. The stigma attached to a homosexual orientation in our society (which may be lessening) can be very destructive and can be echoed in health settings.

Trigger

Take some time to think about your own gender identity and sexual orientation. Don't feel you have to do this exercise – but if you feel ready for it, ask yourself the following questions:

- What is my gender identity and sexual orientation?
- Have these changed at all over time? If so, what caused that change?
- Do I know people whose sexual orientation is different from my own?
- How did I find out about their sexual orientation? How does it make me feel?
- Do I know anyone who has changed their gender identity? What was my reaction?

There are no 'right' answers to any of these questions. However, reflecting on our own experiences and feelings may help us to become more empathetic to the people we meet, both professionally and socially.

Frameworks of sexuality

Midwives are concerned with sexuality because sexual acts involving the sexual/reproductive organs of a man and a woman are involved in conception and thus related to pregnancy and childbirth. This is sexuality at the biological level.

However it is clear, after a moment's thought, that most contemporary sexual acts, even between a man and a woman, and involving penile-vaginal intercourse, are not intended to result in reproduction. Most sexual acts, with or without contraception, are engaged in for reasons other than the desire to conceive a child. These can include pleasure, intimacy, to express love, to conform to social norms, as a duty, as a means of feeling adult/normal/loved, and for money, due to coercion or violence and so on.

It should be becoming clear that sexuality is not just biological, but psychological, emotional, relational and social. Sexuality is constructed, thought about and regulated in various frameworks of meaning. These include a legal framework, a moral framework, a social-cultural framework, a psychological framework and a medical framework.

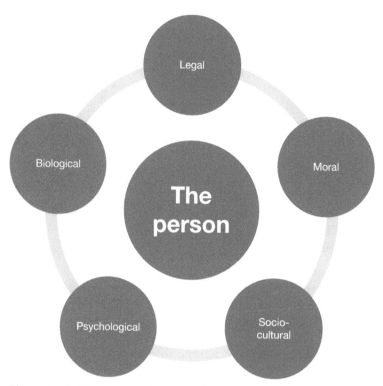

Figure 11.1 The various frameworks associated with sexuality

Legal aspects of sexuality

In the UK this refers mostly to age of consent, sexual violence, sexual grooming, incest and prostitution. In other countries specific acts or practices may be included e.g. adultery, fornication and anal intercourse.

Trigger

In the UK there are certain sexual acts and practices that are illegal and will involve the police and criminal justice system if discovered. Seek out human and material recourses to help you identify these sexual acts and practices.

As a midwife you may find yourself caring for a woman while having to consider the legal aspects of sexuality as well. For example the age of consent to sexual intercourse in the UK is 16. If you are caring for a pregnant 14 year old girl, you will have to consider aspects of safeguarding, because pregnancy in a child under the age of sexual consent implies that an illegal act has been committed. Caring for a woman who discloses domestic violence or sexual abuse will also bring a legal framework into play.

Biological framework of sexuality

This is the framework with which most health professionals are familiar and comfortable. Within the biological framework emphasis is usually placed on reproduction but sexually transmitted infections are also relevant, as are diseases or dysfunctions of reproductive or sexual organs. Within midwifery, difficulties of reproduction itself, infertility and the effect of sexually transmitted infections upon pregnancy or conception are biological aspects of sexuality.

Moral and religious framework of sexuality

Certain sexual practices, orientations or timings may be considered wrong or sinful by society as a whole or more likely by parts of society, and by some religious or ethnic groups.

The reproductive decisions and attitudes of the women in your care may be considered in terms of religious teaching or understanding. Sometimes sexual infection or dysfunction may be considered as punishment (or self-punishment). Even in a non-religious context most of us have strong ideas of what we consider morally acceptable or unacceptable in terms of sexual behaviour. As a midwife, your own personal and wider society's moral or religious frameworks, in which sexuality is framed, will influence your own feelings and those of the women you care for. Recognising and respecting both your own moral attitudes and those of the women in your care, while maintaining a non-judgemental and non-discriminatory practice, can be difficult and takes experience and self-reflection.

Psychological framework of sexuality

The most well-known psychological framework in which sexuality is considered is Freudian psychoanalysis. We shall look at this is more depth in the section that considers theories of sexuality. For the moment it is worth noting that sexuality is not thought of as a purely physical act or need but is recognised to have psychological and emotional aspects and to be closely related to self-identity. If someone is unable to express aspects of their sexual feelings, or perform aspects of what they believe to be their sexual role, this can affect self-esteem and cause great distress. For example, men with erectile difficulties and women unable to conceive or to achieve orgasm often suffer psychological harm.

When people consider sex and sexuality they often slide between frameworks of meaning. Sometimes biological understandings are used to reinforce other frameworks, such as moral and legal frameworks e.g. an aspect of sexuality may be considered wrong because it is unhealthy (promiscuity), or considered illegal because it is 'unnatural' or unrelated to reproduction (anal sex, oral sex, homosexuality).

But moral frameworks can also influence biological understanding e.g. an aspect of sexuality considered to be morally 'wrong' was also considered to be a sign of illness (homosexuality) or to cause illness (masturbation in the nineteenth century). It is important to think about the various frameworks of sexuality and consider which ones are active or pertinent to the context in which midwifery is being practiced.

Theories of sexuality

Evolutionary

Evolutionary explanations for sexuality focus on the need for reproduction in order to maintain the species. This theoretical view is necessarily reductionist, in that it 'brackets out' non-biological and non- reproductive aspects of sexuality, and focuses on those acts and behaviours that lead to conception and pregnancy. This approach is useful but most couples experience sexuality in much broader terms. Psychological and relational aspects of sexuality such as of emotion, commitment and relationship building are omitted. An evolutionary approach also excludes the profound effect that cultural norms and, to a lesser extent, legal frameworks, can have on how sexuality is expressed and experienced.

Post-structuralist

The post-structuralist approach to sexuality, in contrast to the evolutionary approach, is very concerned with how social and cultural factors shape, constrain and create what we call 'sexuality'. Its most famous proponent is the social theorist Michel Foucault who famously argued that sexuality, sexual feelings, sexual acts and sexual identities are not essentially biological but socially created: 'sex is the most speculative, most ideal and most internal element in a deployment of sexuality organised by power in its grip on bodies and their materialities, their forces, energies, sensations and pleasures' (Foucault, 1998: 155).

On a broader level post-structuralist approaches to sexuality argue that what we consider 'normal' and 'abnormal' in terms of sexuality is mostly the result of cultural norms and social negotiation. For instance, what we would now call child marriage and under-age sexual intercourse was commonplace and acceptable in earlier centuries, and is still acceptable in some parts of the world. Powerful actors in the negotiation of what is normal and acceptable are religious authorities, scientific and medical authorities and governmental authorities. Certain sexual practices, sexual relationships and even sexual positions can be deemed immoral or unhealthy, and therefore socially unacceptable. However the post-structuralist approach also recognises that 'top-down' authority has limited effect. The intimate, micro-relations between people will also determine how sexuality is constructed. An example of this is the debate around breastfeeding in public. Medical authorities are strongly in favour of breastfeeding, and religious authorities are mostly silent on the matter, but whether or not a woman feels she can breastfeed in a public space is more often decided by the reactions of those who encounter her there. If at a micro-social level, e.g. in a café, most social participants view breasts as sexual organs, not nutritional organs, then breastfeeding may be constructed as a sexual act, and therefore draw opprobrium. This displeasure and disapproval will have a powerful constraining effect on a woman who wants to breastfeed, and may dissuade her on that occasion or perhaps permanently. Post-structuralist approaches also recognise the enormous effect of language upon social norms. This is why debates about terms such as 'prostitutes v. sex workers' have significance and why minority groups will sometimes appropriate derogatory terms used against them, and subvert them to remove their stigmatising power.

The idea that governance and sanction can operate between individuals makes it important for health professionals to reflect upon and understand their own views on sexuality, and consider how their actions may convey those views and constrain or enable the actions, questions and decisions of the women for whom they care. The power inherent in language is important when considering the wording of official forms, which can exclude people in non-traditional family structures and the way in which questions may be put to a pregnant woman, which may inadvertently cause offence or distress.

Psychoanalytical

Psychoanalytical theories of sexuality are varied, but most, including classical Freudian psychoanalytical theory, view sexual behaviour as originating from a primary sexual drive, which it names 'libido'. Psychoanalytical views of sexuality share some features of post-structuralist views, in as much as they do not see sexual behaviour as primarily reproductive in either origin or intent. For Freud, the young child was 'polymorphously perverse', deriving pleasure from varied physical sensations and sources, including the mouth, the anus and the clitoris or penis. The aim of the libido is to seek a discharge for sexual excitement, and any 'object' can be used for this, including parts of the body, parts of another person's body, and other people or inanimate objects. Where psychoanalytical theory agrees with evolutionary theory is that Freud argued that the polymorphously perverse character of the young child is eventually, as a result of many trials, including the famous Oedipal crisis, 'organised' into mature genital sexuality, with the outcome of heterosexual, reproductive intercourse. However Freud was also clear that other sexual preferences and behaviours were not completely eliminated but remained unconscious and influential, and that the ultimate organisation of sexuality into heterosexual reproductive activity was in large part due to parental, social and educational constraints. Where the psychoanalytical model is most informative for midwifery practice is arguably in its insight that sexuality is always complex and subject to unconscious feelings of guilt, unconscious desires and multiple overlaid meanings. Psychoanalytical theory strongly emphasises that sexuality is a fundamental part of humanity and has influences far beyond genital, sexual activity.

Sexuality and midwifery practice

Sexuality impinges upon midwifery practice in a number of ways. Most obviously and universally, the women for whom midwives care will have sexual desires and sexual relationships that are very likely to be affected by childbirth (von Sydow, 1999). While this is not the primary focus of midwifery care, the midwife is well placed to advise of these sensitive issues because of the close and trusting relationship she will develop with the woman for whom she cares.

In some cases the sexuality of pregnant women will be of a minority type i.e. the woman may identify as lesbian and/or have a female partner. While this is not relevant to the kind of physical care the woman will need, the midwife's response and attitude towards this will have a powerful effect upon the supportive, psychological and emotional care that she can give the couple (Dibley, 2009; Hayman et al., 2013; Rondahl et al., 2009; Spidsberg, 2007). Some women will have experienced sexual violence or sexual abuse in their lives (Wijma et al., 2003). This may have an effect on their experience of midwifery care, and in some cases it may be more difficult for the woman to fully trust the care she is given.

Application to practice

Have a look at the information leaflets or websites produced by your employer that are available to women and their partners during pregnancy and after the birth. These may include a whole range of information including: screening in pregnancy; place of birth; breastfeeding etc. Using the knowledge gained from this chapter, consider the following:

- How inclusive is the language in these leaflets? Could it be improved, and if so, how?
- How inclusive are the images? For example, is there at least one photo of two women sitting together? An image like this will go unnoticed by people who are heterosexual, but sends out an important message to lesbian couples that they are acknowledged and affirmed.
- Do any of the leaflets acknowledge that sexual feelings may change during or after birth?
- Do any of the leaflets give contact details for support groups, such as the government website (http://thisisabuse.direct.gov.uk/need-help) or the mental health charity Mind (www.mind.org.uk)

Make a note of any aspects of these leaflets and websites that could be improved. Once you have done that, make an appointment with a colleague (for example, a consultant midwife) involved in the design and production of these. Aim to have three to five constructive suggestions, and make it clear that you would like to be involved in ongoing development of the information.

Sexuality, pregnancy and childbirth

The effect of pregnancy and childbirth upon sexuality and sexual behaviour is an area about which many midwives feel they lack knowledge. Research that has been carried out into the subject provides an evidence base for advice, but it remains an under-researched area.

A meta-analysis of 59 research studies (von Sydow, 1999) found that, methodologically, conceptual reductionism was common (i.e. sexuality = intercourse), and that the experiences of male partners and the non-sexual aspects of relationships were often neglected in research studies. It is therefore important to bear in mind that sexuality and sexual expression can take forms other than 'penis-in-vagina' intercourse, and to take into account factors that are, strictly speaking, non-sexual such as financial and social strains, cultural expectations and relationship satisfaction.

Von Sydow's meta-analysis found that sexual interest and coital activity in both men and women decreases in the third trimester, but also found that there was a great deal of variation between individuals (von Sydow, 1999: 35). Men showed more sexual initiative than female partners before, during and after pregnancy, and female sexual activity was often motivated by a concern for the male partner (von Sydow, 1999: 36). The average time from birth to first intercourse was six to eight weeks in the United Kingdom and United States, and almost all couple had resumed intercourse by the third month (95 per cent). For most couples frequency of sexual intercourse was reduced in the first year after birth, compared to pre-pregnancy rates. Sexual problems post-birth were reported commonly, with only 14 per cent of women and 12 per cent of men reporting no problems (von Sydow, 1999: 37). These included dyspareunia (painful intercourse) in more than half of women, with 22 per cent still reporting this at 13 months, although 12 per cent of women reported this symptom before pregnancy.

In the long term, the effect of pregnancy and childbirth on sexual relationships varied with one third of couples reporting a worsening of sexual relationship at three to four years but 20 per cent of women reporting an intensification of their sexual lives. Women also reported intense physical pleasure and sexual feelings during breastfeeding, with many feeling guilty about this (von Sydow, 1999: 39).

Couples reported that they would have liked to have received more information about bodily changes and sexual relationships post-partum, and that the information received was entirely focused on full intercourse and often restrictive, for example, advising delaying resumption of intercourse until the lochia had stopped and menstruation had resumed (von Sydow, 1999: 38). Interestingly the paper suggests that the women in the studies who asked their gynaecologists for advice about sex during pregnancy often received only advice about avoiding or limiting sex, in specific circumstances, whereas books, birth preparation courses and advice from female friends had a positive effect on sexual enjoyment in pregnancy.

Some men reported worrying that the fetus could be hurt during intercourse. Interestingly painful or complicated births did not reduce post-partum sexual activity or enjoyment, although women in the studies who had experienced perineal lacerations sometimes reported a delay in resumption of sexual activity. However complicated and painful birth experiences did reduce tenderness between partners in the post-partum period.

Depressed mood during pregnancy had a negative effect on sexual enjoyment and activity and the perceived tenderness of the partner (von Sydow, 1999: 40). Lastly the meta-analysis found that if partners are enjoyably sexually active during pregnancy, the relationship between them is better evaluated post-partum and more stable three years later.

The author of the review noted the extreme inter-individual variability of many of the findings and suggested that more research is needed on biographical and partnership factors. She also suggested that sexual partners' post-partum adjustment to parenthood is much more complex than the mother's physical adaptation to pregnancy and childbirth, in terms of the effect on sexuality.

A more recent qualitative study, in which women participated in focus groups between 3 and 24 months after delivery, found that some women were distressed at the changes to their bodies following pregnancy, and that this decreased sexual interest (Olsson et al., 2005). Women reported that the tiredness and busyness associated with caring for a new baby made sex less of a priority, and they also reported a discordance of desire with their male partners. The women expressed a need for reassurance about their physical health and the state of their post-partum bodies, and hoped that the post-natal review would provide this. They also expressed a need for more time to be spent on discussing aspects of their sexual life, and felt that a second post-natal appointment at four to five months might be a more appropriate time to do this.

Father's experiences

MacAdam et al. (2011), in a qualitative study of the experiences of 12 fathers interviewed 6–13 months after the birth of their baby, found that fathers reported a lack of reciprocation with regard to sex from their female partners. Most accepted this and saw it as a temporary state of affairs. Fathers also commented that caring for the child and caring for their partner brought about new ways of expressing tenderness and intimacy that did not involve intercourse, and they tended to prioritise the relationship with their partner at that point in parenthood.

Couple's relationship

The birth of a first baby may make a significant change to a couple's relationship and can affect its quality. A systematic review of seven primary research papers found that couples reported a loss of intimacy and difficulties with communication (Bateman and Bharj, 2009). The review's authors suggested that midwives were well placed to address some of these problems.

Midwives' views

Olsson et al. (2011) looked at the views of midwives on offering advice on sexuality to women at the post-natal check-up. They found that midwives complained of lack of time, and also a fear that they would not know how to advise once a woman started to confide about sexual problems. Sometimes advice on contraception, pelvic floor exercises or a vaginal examination opened the way for a discussion of the woman's sexual experience since the birth of her baby. The authors noted that the return to having sexual intercourse after childbirth partly depended upon cultural norms, and that midwives need to reflect upon their own unacknowledged cultural expectations because of the powerful situation in which they were positioned with regard to defining 'normal' behaviour.

The available evidence suggests that pregnancy and childbirth has a significant effect on sexuality and sexual relations for nearly every couple, but that their effects can be very varied. It is clear that most women would welcome some advice or reassurance about sexual matters both during and after pregnancy. Some reduction in sexual activity both in late pregnancy and post-natally is usual but most couples will resume full intercourse by the time the baby is three months old. Tiredness, busyness, communication difficulties and loss of intimacy can be regarded as being as important in regard to a couple's sexual relationship as any physical changes to the woman's body caused by pregnancy and birth.

Implications for midwives

Midwives should be prepared to discuss sex and sexual relationships with women in their care. Focusing only on the resumption of full sexual intercourse after childbirth may be too restrictive and including advice on topics such as affection, intimacy, communication and making time for one another is likely to be helpful. Midwives should be aware of the variation in experience for couples around sexual activity, so that they can reassure women and their partners, but should also be able to suggest referral or self-referral to alternative sources of advice, if they feel that a couple have difficulties that are beyond the limits of their own competency.

Trigger

To stimulate your thoughts and feelings about sexuality within the sphere of midwifery practice, read this article written by Meg Taylor in 1994:

http://midwifery.megtaylor.co.uk/index.php?option=com_content&view=article&id=9:labour-and-sexuality&catid=1:midwifery&Itemid=2

How do you feel about what Meg has written? Have you ever witnessed women in labour making noises similar to orgasm? If so, how did you feel and how did you react? Did you try to encourage the woman to be quiet? And if so, why?

Same sex parenting

Although, within a biological framework, conception requires male and female gametes, social parenting is aspired to and accomplished by many lesbian couples, and, to a lesser extent, gay male couples.

There are no figures for numbers of lesbians embarking on pregnancy, and estimating the proportion of lesbian and gay people in the general population is notoriously difficult. In the most recent National Survey of Sexual Attitudes and Lifestyles (NATSAL) some 5 per cent of men and 8 per cent of women between 16 and 44 years reported 'ever' having had a same sex experience with genital contact (NATSAL, 2013). The estimated number of same sex households in England and Wales in 2010 was between 68,000 and 88,000 (Ross et al., 2011). Numbers of women who self-identify as lesbian and also experience pregnancy will be fewer. Nonetheless midwives in the course of their career today are likely to encounter lesbian mothers and their female partners.

An awareness of the various aspects of sexuality and sexual orientation is useful because midwives will have their own views and experiences of lesbian sexuality and of same sex parents that may influence the care that they deliver. There will also be lesbian midwives who are delivering care, to heterosexual and lesbian parents.

Small qualitative studies of the experiences of lesbian couples during midwifery care have been carried out in the UK, Australia, Norway and Sweden. These give some insight into the care that lesbian woman have experienced while being cared for by midwives.

Dibley (2009) interviewed ten lesbian women about their experiences of midwifery care in the UK, and found that they reported a variety of experiences from positive to neutral to openly hostile. They reported a 'heterosexist' assumption, in that midwives assumed that these women were heterosexual until they were corrected. This placed an onus upon the lesbian women to reveal their sexuality explicitly, which could be a stressful experience, since they were not sure of the reaction that they would receive. In some cases the paperwork and documentation that needed to be completed was phrased in a manner that assumed the partner of the woman would be male. Negative experiences reported by the women included one midwife allegedly refusing to care for the couple during a home delivery, and another preventing another couple from attending antenatal classes. Other lesbian women reported positive, supportive experiences from their midwives and still others described their experience as neither good nor bad.

Hayman et al. (2013) report similar experiences from a larger qualitative study of 15 lesbian couples in Australia. They also reported heterosexist assumptions, exclusion (excluding female partners from various procedures) and inappropriate questioning (particularly with regard to standard documentation). The authors note that:

> the passage to motherhood can be particularly demanding for lesbian mothers as they navigate the usual challenges of motherhood alongside the challenges of birthing and raising children in a heteronormative social context that can

have disabling features such as stigmatisation, discrimination and homophobia. (Hayman et al., 2013: 121)

The authors advocate the assumption of a 'culturally sensitive' practice in midwifery, including the culture of same sex couples.

Spidsberg (2007) narrates the experiences of six lesbian couples in Norway, who reported both caring situations and some less-caring situations while experiencing maternity care. At times these couples were unsure if their sexuality was the cause of the poor care they were receiving. She also reports that lesbian couples felt responsible for managing interaction in the face of uncertainty and anxiety on the part of healthcare providers. Rondhal et al. (2009) interviewed ten lesbian mothers who, despite largely positive experiences, experienced an assumption of heterosexuality, which was embarrassing for them and made them anxious about revealing their sexuality.

Spidsberg and Sorlie (2012) carried out a descriptive study of the experience of midwives dealing with lesbian parents in Norway. They found that midwives described caring for lesbian couples as 'unproblematic' but also reported some ambivalences and anxiety, sometimes arising from personal attitudes to homosexuality, and sometimes arising from worry about appearing inadvertently judgemental or homophobic. They described the relationships between lesbian couples as 'strong and caring' but recognised that co-mothers had different roles and needs to fathers.

Finally Mander and Page (2012) discuss the experience of lesbian and gay midwives. Their literature search revealed an assumption of heterosexuality and the need to 'come out' repeatedly. They also discuss the dilemma of whether or not a lesbian midwife discloses her sexuality to the women for whom she cares. Overall they found that lesbian midwives were largely invisible in the workforce in the UK, which was compared unfavourably to the situation in other countries and with regards to lesbian and gay doctors and nurses.

There is very little research in this area but some qualitative studies reveal that the experience of lesbian mothers varies but also that some persistent points of difficulty are highlighted again and again. These are heterosexist assumptions, particularly those embedded in standard paperwork, and anxiety felt by lesbian mothers about when and whether to 'come out' to midwifery and other staff. There are also reports of anxiety and discomfort experienced by staff and women in their care, because of the fear of discrimination and/or judgemental attitudes (on the part of lesbian women) or the fear of appearing judgmental or insensitive (on the part of staff) and the need to constantly negotiate this.

Implications for midwives

As a minimum midwives should be aware that not every woman in their care will have a male sexual partner or consider herself to be heterosexual. Inclusive and sensitive opening questions, when meeting a woman for the first time, will help lesbian women to feel welcome and less anxious about 'coming out' to staff. Discrimination on the grounds of sexual orientation is both unprofessional and, in the UK, illegal.

The effect of sexual abuse upon pregnancy, childbirth and midwifery

Pregnant and post-natal women may experience or have experienced sexual abuse or violence, either in their adult relationships or as children. This may affect how they experience their pregnancies and the care they receive. In a cross-sectional study involving 3,641 gynaecology patients in five Nordic countries, Wijma et al. (2003) found a lifetime prevalence of sexual abuse of between 17 and 30 per cent. This suggests that a significant number of women in the care of midwives will have experienced sexual abuse. This may affect their experience of examination, especially vaginal examination, during routine care. Many healthcare professionals are unsure about raising the issue of sexual abuse, due to a lack of training, lack of experience or a lack of organisational support, including time, to allow the issue to be discussed (Wendt et al., 2011). Wendt et al. (2007) found that 72 per cent of young women attending for cervical smears would find questions about sexual abuse acceptable, although the majority had not been asked such questions. Studies with pregnant women (Stensson et al., 2001) and women attending emergency departments (Kramer et al., 2004) have shown that around 80 per cent find questions from clinicians about violence, including sexual violence, acceptable.

Child sexual abuse is a subset of sexual violence. Montgomery (2013) found that women who had experienced child sexual abuse (CSA) could experience flash backs and reminders of the abusive situation during routine antenatal care. Feeling 'safe' during antenatal care involved not being put in situations that reminded them of their abusive experiences. Enabling women to retain control of what was happening to them and forging positive and trusting relationships with staff could help women negotiate the difficulties of maternity care and childbirth.

Rhodes and Hutchinson (1994) identified four labouring styles that may be adopted by women who had experienced CSA. They termed these 'fighting', 'taking control', 'surrendering' and 'retreating'. Recognising these styles may help midwives manage an otherwise difficult labouring situation. Loss of control during labour can be particularly difficult for women who have experienced CSA because of the association with the loss of control during abuse. Dissociation from the present situation was often reported as a coping style.

The experience of childbirth and perinatal care can evoke traumatic associations for those who experience or have experienced sexual abuse. The incidence of women receiving pregnancy care who have experienced sexual abuse is unknown but is likely to be much higher than commonly assumed. Loss of control is a difficult situation for such women to handle and can result in a variety of coping styles that may seem puzzling or difficult for staff.

Implications for midwives

Midwives should be aware that a small but significant proportion of women for whom they care have experienced or will be experiencing sexual abuse or violence. This may affect the way they behave during antenatal care and childbirth. Clarke and Smythe (2011) have suggested adopting a form of 'universal precautions' to reduce the risk of women, who may have an undisclosed history of sexual abuse, feeling retraumatised by their midwifery care. These include gaining explicit and continuing consent for all procedures (including examination of the baby), clear explanations and the avoidance of 'routine' examinations or procedures if they are unnecessary.

Application to practice

This chapter illustrates many ways in which midwives can reflect on the subject of sexuality and use this knowledge to improve their own practice. However, this cannot be done in isolation. In order to provide effective, holistic and compassionate care, it is important to work with colleagues in other fields. Here are some suggestions:

- Make contact with your local sexual health services. Find out what psychosexual counselling services are available locally, and go and talk to the people who are involved. Ask them about referrals that relate to pregnancy, labour or childbearing. What sort of issues emerge? How do these reflect on clinical practice. Talk to your senior colleagues about setting up a joint meeting or seminar on sharing best practice.
- Make contact with a local LGBT (lesbian, gay, bisexual and trans) support group. Ask them if they could give some advice and ideas for ensuring that the maternity services meet the needs of their users. Talk to your senior colleagues about putting these ideas in to practice.

Conclusion

This chapter has introduced the varied and at times contradictory ways in which sexuality has been theorised, and how these differing frameworks can impact on midwifery practice. It explored in some detail the issues of sexuality in the context of pregnancy and labour and invited you to consider your own experiences in this area. It has discussed the issue of caring for lesbian women and asked you to consider your experiences and views relating to your own sexual orientation and the sexual orientation of other people. Lastly it has looked at the evidence for the effects of child sexual abuse and/or sexual violence and how this may impact on the relationship between the midwife and the woman for whom she is caring.

Considering and reflecting upon aspects of sexuality as they are encountered in midwifery practice provides an opportunity to develop a responsive and informed midwifery practice in this area. Recognising the needs of lesbian mothers and their partners, and ensuring that heterosexist assumptions do not endure, will lead to an inclusive and non-stigmatising professional environment. Similarly recognising the difficulties that experiences of violence, sexual violence or child sexual abuse can cause for women who are giving birth, and for the midwives who care for them, creates opportunities for increased sensitivity and the application of precautionary practice that takes steps to allow women to remain in control. Applying these concepts universally may reduce the chances of pregnancy and birth becoming traumatic experiences, even for those women for whom disclosure of sexual violence or abuse does not take place. Lastly, by becoming more informed and confident about giving advice on sexual feelings and sexual relationships during pregnancy and post-natally, midwives are well placed to advise women struggling with these issues, or to sign post them to further sources of help.

References

Bateman, L. and Bharj, K. 2009. The Impact of the first child on the couple's relationship. *Evidence based Midwifery* 7 (1) pp. 16–23

Clarke, E. and Smythe, L. 2011. The effects of child sexual abuse on labour and birthing: an exploration to assist midwives. *New Zealand College of Midwives Journal* 45 pp. 21–24

Dibley, L.B. 2009. Experiences of lesbian parents in the UK: interactions with midwives. *Evidence Based Midwifery* 7 (3) pp. 94–100

Foucault, M. 1998.*The History of Sexuality Vol. 1.* London: Penguin

Hayman, B., Wilkes, L., Halcomb, E. and Jackson, D. 2013. Marginalised mothers: lesbian women negotiating heteronormative healthcare services. *Contemporary Nurse* 44 (1) pp. 120–127

Kramer, A, Lorenzon, D and Mueller, G. 2004. Prevalence of intimate partner violence and health implications for women using emergency departments and primary care clinics. *Women's Health Issues* 14 pp. 19–29.

MacAdam, R., Huuva, E. and Bertero, C. 2011. Father's experiences after having a child: sexuality becomes tailored according to circumstances. *Midwifery* 27 e149–e155

Mander, R. and Page, M. 2012. Midwifery and the LBGT midwife. *Midwifery* 28 pp. 9–13

Montgomery, E. 2013. Feeling safe: a meta-synthesis of the maternity care needs of women who were sexually abused in childhood. *Birth* 40 (2) pp. 88–95

NATSAL (National Survey of Sexual Attitudes and Lifestyles) 2013. Sexual attitudes and lifestyles in Britain: highlights from Natsal-3. Online at [http://www.natsal.ac.uk/media/823260/natsal_findings_final.pdf]

Olsson, A.,Lundqvist, M., Faxelid, E. and Nissen, E. 2005 Women's thoughts about sexual life after childbirth. *Scandinavian Journal of Caring Sciences* 19 pp. 381–387

Olsson, A., Robertson, E., Falk, K. and Nissen, E. 2011. Assessing women's sexual life after childbirth: the role of the postnatal check. *Midwifery* 27 (2), pp. 195 –202

Rhodes, N. and Hutchinson, S. 1994. Labour experiences of childhood sexual abuse survivors. *Birth* 21 (4) pp. 26–39

Rondhal, G., Bruhner, E. and Lindhe, J. 2009. Heteronormative communication with lesbian families in antenatal care, childbirth and post natal care. *Journal of Advanced Nursing* 65 (11) pp. 2337–2344

Ross, H. Gask, K. and Berringham, A. 2011. Civil partnerships five years on. *Population Trends* No. 145, Autumn

Spidsberg, B.D. 2007 Vulnerable and strong: lesbian women encountering maternity care. *Journal of Advanced Nursing* 60 (5) pp. 478–486

Spidsberg, B. D. and Sorlie, V. 2012. An expression of love: midwives' experiences in the encounter with lesbian woman and their partners. *Journal of Advanced Nursing* 68 (4) pp. 796–805

Stensson, K.,Saarinen, H., Heimer G. et al.2001.Women's attitudes to being asked about exposure to violence. *Midwifery*, 17 (2001), pp. 2–10

von Sydow, K. 1999. Sexuality during pregnancy and after childbirth: a meta-content analysis of 59 studies. *Journal of Psychosomatic Research* 47 (1) pp. 27–49.

Wendt, E.K., Hildingh, C.I., Lidell, E.A., Westerståhl, A.K.E., Baigi, A. and Marklund, B.R.G. 2007. Young women's sexual health and their views on dialogue with health professionals. *Acta Obstetrica et Gynecologica Scandinavia* 86 pp. 590–595

Wendt, E.K., Lidell, E.A., Marklund, B.R.G., Hildingh, C.I. and Westerståhl, A.K.E. 2011. Possibilities for dialogue on sexuality and sexual abuse – midwives' and clinician's experiences. *Midwifery* 27 (3) pp. 539–546

Wijma, B., Schei, B., Swahnberg, K., Hilden, M., Offerdal, K., Pikarinen, U., Sidenius, K., Steingrimsdottir, T., Stoum, H. and Halmesmäki, E. 2003. Emotional, physical, and sexual abuse in patients visiting gynaecology clinics: a Nordic cross-sectional study. *Lancet* 361 pp. 2107–13

Glossary

Advocacy within the context of midwifery seeks to defend and safeguard women's rights and ensure that they and their families have their voice heard and are able to access information and services and have the opportunity to fully explore their options and choices

Aetiology the cause or set of causes for a condition

Attachment the affectional tie that forms between the child and another, usually the parent or carer

Autonomy refers to the capacity for self-determination and/or self-governance

Biases are influences that have the potential to distort the findings of a study and affect the internal validity of a study

Biomedicine (allopathic medicine; western medicine; scientific medicine) is ethnomedicine of industrialised societies with core values based on science and technology

Blues/baby blues a frequently observed phenomenon, usually occurring in the first week postpartum and characterised by emotional lability

Bonding a mother's or father's emotional connection to their baby

Bourgeoisie a term used by Karl Marx and those influenced by him to denote those who belonged to the ruling classes within a capitalist society and who owned the majority of the means of production

Cognitive involving conscious mental activities, for example thinking, learning and remembering

Collective conscience a term used in sociology to refer to the shared beliefs and moral principles that function as a unifying force within society

Conflict theory a term used within sociology to highlight the role of oppression and power in producing social order

Consensus theory used within sociology emphasising the importance of the role of the collective conscience and having shared values to ensure stability, social order and regulation within society

Consultant midwife this role was developed as a means of ensuring clinical expertise and leadership on both a strategic and clinical level. The key domains of the consultant midwife role are:

- expert practice
- professional leadership and consultancy

- education, training and development
- practice and service development
- research and evaluation

Constructivism is a paradigm or worldview that emphasises that learning is an active process whereby knowledge and meaning is constructed through our interaction with the social world

Control refers to the language, views, morals, norms, customs, roles, knowledge and skills that make up the way of life within any society

Critical theory provides a specific interpretation of Marxist philosophy and similarly is concerned with critiquing and changing society as a whole

Deductive reasoning is sometimes referred to as a 'top-down approach'; this is where the researcher works from having a general theory or hypothesis and seeks to reach a specific conclusion whereby they can reject or confirm their initial theory or hypothesis

Discourse a way of communicating that reveals ways of thinking and producing meaning

Empiricism is a theory that knowledge can only be obtained through sensory experience

Empower within midwifery means to engender and facilitate an individual or group's control and influence

Epistemology is a theory of knowledge or the branch of philosophy that studies the nature of knowledge, in particular its foundations, scope and validity

Ethnography is the systematic study and interpretation of peoples and cultures. It is designed to explore cultural phenomena where the researcher observes society from the point of view of the subject of the study

Ethnomethodology is a branch of interpretative sociological inquiry and qualitative research method that aims to explore how people make sense of their social activities and interactions

Evidence-based practice is the thorough, overt and judicious use of current best evidence helping midwives make decisions about the care of individual women

External validity refers to the extent to which the study findings can be generalised to other settings

Functionalism is a broad sociological theory that views society as being made up of different parts or relationships that are all in some way related. This is often referred to as structural theory or structural functionalism

Generalisability refers to the degree to which the findings of the research study can be extrapolated to the population outside of the study

Hermeneutic approach to social study is the interpretation of meanings of social actions of participants

Iatrogenesis refers to any adverse consequence that result from medical treatment or intervention

Inductive reasoning is sometimes referred to as a 'bottom-up approach'; this is where theories are generated from specific observations and the detection of themes and patterns within the data

Intellectual pluralism put simply means that no particular view of reality or perspective can account for all the phenomena of life

Internal validity refers to the extent to which the experimental treatment is responsible for the observed effects (rather than uncontrolled factors or variables)

Interpretative approach concentrates on the meanings people associate to their social world and endeavours to demonstrate how reality is constructed by people themselves in their daily lives

Leadership refers to the process of leading an organisation, group or individuals

Macro perspective refers to an approach where social processes and systems are analysed on a large scale or in their entirety

Marxism refers to a broad sociological theory that focuses on or has its origins in the work of Karl Marx and broadly speaking focuses on the economic structure within society and the conflicts between those that have material wealth and those who do not

Maternity service liaison committees are made up of a group of people who are involved in planning, providing and receiving maternity care, and who advise on developments in local maternity services and monitor progress towards agreed standards so that all parents profit from improvements in care

Medicalised or medicalisation means to treat something as a medical problem

Methodology refers to a system of general principles or rules from which specific methods or procedures may be derived to inform those who are in sociological research inquiry

Micro perspective refers to an approach where social systems and processes are analysed on a smaller scale taking into account the small-scale interaction that occurs between individuals

Midwifery-led care refers to when midwives are the lead professionals in planning and implementing maternity care in partnership with women

Naturalised childbirth is generally based on the belief that pregnancy and birth is a normal physiological process and support and coping strategies are focused on supporting these physiological processes and optimising the opportunity for normal birth

Occupational jurisdiction within this context refers to the power right for one professional group to exercise their authority and expertise

Ontology used within research to refer to the nature of reality and existence

Operational definition used to clearly define the details of the process, measures and variables are within the scientific approach to research

Organisational culture refers to a shared set of understandings, values and beliefs related to a particular occupation

Paradigm a term used within research theory to describe a particular perspective or way of looking at things

Phenomenology a branch of interpretative sociological inquiry and qualitative research method that aims to explore the lived experiences of individuals

Phobia an extreme or irrational fear of, or aversion to, something

Positivist discourse is a way of thinking developed by Auguste Comte. It is a philosophical system recognising only that which can be scientifically verified or which is capable of logical or mathematical proof, and therefore rejecting metaphysics and theism. Randomised controlled trials are an example of a research method that would be described as positivist in nature

Positivist theory Positivism is the philosophy of science that information derived from logical and mathematical treatments is the exclusive source of all authoritative knowledge and that there is valid knowledge only in this derived knowledge. Intuitive knowledge is rejected

Postnatal depression is depression suffered by a mother following childbirth

Proletariat a term used within Marxist theory of capitalist societies to denote those that belonged to the working classes and who were exploited by those who owned the means of production, namely the bourgeoisie

Psychoanalyst a therapist who uses a system of psychological theory and therapy involving investigation of personality by exploring both conscious and unconscious elements in the mind

Psychosis a severe mental disorder in which impaired thought and emotions cause loss of contact with external reality

Psychotic a person suffering from psychosis (see also psychosis)

Puerperal psychosis the sudden onset of psychotic symptoms following childbirth

Puerperium the period of about six weeks after childbirth during which the mother's reproductive organs return to their original non-pregnant condition

Qualitative research uses research methods that result in a narrative descriptive account and involves collecting and/or working with text, images or sounds

Quantitative research uses research methods that result in collecting numerical data and analysed mathematically usually through statistical analysis

Reductionist is a philosophical position that states that the nature of complex processes and systems can be understood by reducing them to their individual components or parts

Reflexivity a term used to take account of the potential imprint of the researcher upon the qualitative research process and acknowledges that it is impossible to separate the researcher from the research study

Reliability refers to the consistency with which an instrument measures what it is designed to measure

Research methods refer to the stages, procedures and strategies for collecting and analysing data within a research investigation

Sanctions are the rewards and punishments by which social control is achieved and conformity to norms and values enforced. These may be positive sanctions (rewards of various kinds) or negative sanctions (types of punishment)

Scientific method refers to a research process that incorporates a set of systematic procedures for acquiring empirical data and is associated with the positivistic paradigm

Social action theory is concerned with meaning and assumes that humans vary their actions in accordance with social contexts and emphasises the ability of individuals to exercise control over their own actions

Socialisation the process of learning the culture of any given society

Social or cultural system organisations with shared ideas, concepts, rules and meanings that underlie and are expressed in the ways that humans interact

Structuration is a sociological theory that focuses on how societies are sustained by a combination of structure and action

Structural theories a broad sociological theory that views society as being made up of different parts or relationships that are all in some way related. This is often referred to as functionalism or structural functionalism

Symbolic interactionism is a sociological theory that endeavours to explain social behaviour in terms of how people engage with each other via words, gestures and other symbols that have acquired conventional meanings within society

Woman-centred care refers to a philosophy of maternity care that gives priority to the wishes and needs of the user. The core principles of woman-centred care are as follows:

- ensuring women are equal partners in the planning and delivery of maternity care
- ensuring women have informed choice in terms of the options available during pregnancy, labour and the postnatal period
- the provision of continuity of care and formation of transparent, trusting relationships
- ensuring women are empowered and have control over the key decisions affecting the content and progress of their care

Index

Note: **bold** text denotes an illustration, *italics* a table, and the suffix 'g' refers to the Glossary.